INTRODUCTION

Living inside a Disaster Movie?

A young Chinese Doctor, Lin Wen Liang, in a hospital bed, farewells family and friends…

In a deserted Piazza San Marco, a policewoman, wearing a mask, looks at two girls, wearing, themselves too, masks: ornate Columbina masks.

Cristiano Ronaldo on TV wearing a mask…football games will be played behind closed doors.

On Ash Wednesday, during the General Audience in St. Peter's Square, Pope Francis said, "I wish, again, to express my closeness to those who are ill with coronavirus and to health-care workers who are caring for them."

Jackie Chan quarantined after a private party.

Production for the upcoming "Mission: Impossible" movie has been put on hold due to the worldwide coronavirus outbreak. A three-week shoot was set to take place in Venice, Italy, but the country has had a recent surge of the viral disease. The epicenter of the outbreak is in northern Italy, and the number of confirmed cases hit already thousands...

Night and day frantic building... From January 24th to February 3rd Chinese government builds two 1600 beds hospitals at Wuhan City. In just ten days...

Ten villages quarantined in north Italy.

An eleven million people city closed in China. Then sixteen more. Over fifty million people under lockdown...

3700 quarantined in the Diamond Princess.

Closed borders. In Asia. In Europe. In the Middle East...Almost all over the world...

No flights. No trains. Drones chasing those defying lockdown.

Saudi Arabia bans foreign pilgrims from visiting Mecca...

Work goes remote...

Not a Disaster-Hollywood-post-apocalyptic movie. Just everyday news since COVID-19 breakout.

A very good time to remember that the only real enemies Mankind ever faced are IGNORANCE, and his spoiled child, FEAR.

Ignorance and Fear, not disease.

Ignorance and Fear, not hunger.

Ignorance and Fear, not tyrants.

Together, this two ones, I bet, did more harm than any plague...

Imagine: Your Life, free from Ignorance and Fear.

Imagine: Your Family, free from Ignorance and Fear.

Imagine: your Community, free from Ignorance and Fear.

Imagine: The World, free from Ignorance and Fear.

So let's educate ourselves.

Less Ignorance, more Knowledge.

Do not Fear, just Care.

ABOUT THIS BOOK

This book is divided in two chapters:

Chapter One: What you need to Know

Chapter Two: Take Action

In **Chapter One** we will first clarify the meanings of some basic **words** you will find repeatedly on Media. Expressions like Infectious Disease, Virus, Endemic, Epidemic and Pandemic, Ro Value or Basic Reproduction Rate, Mortality Rate, Case Fatality Rate, and Community Spread.

Then we will discuss **facts**: Statistics, Global Death Rates, Viral Pandemics (the Spanish Flu, SARS, MERS and COVID-19), and other human coronaviruses according to the most reliable sources: World Health Organization, and United States Centers for Disease Control.

After that we will **surf the web** for the latest news and trending topics on the Internet about COVID-19 outbreak. COVID-19 and Influenza; COVID-19 Case Fatality Rate (CFR) discussion, COVID-19 Incubation Period and COVID-19 and pets.

In the last section you will find the most complete **TimeLine** of COVID-19 outbreak, since 2019 December the 1st until today. Writing this timeline helped me understand each new incoming piece of information, and I hope it will help you too.

In **Chapter Two: Take Action**, I will share with you some great information to strengthen your Immune System and help protect yourself, your loved ones and your community.

In the Appendices I, II and III you will find World Health Organization and United States Centers for Disease Control recommendations.

Initially a **Third Chapter** called Global Narratives was planned. In that third chapter we would entertain ourselves with the scariest, most worrying and freaking urban myths. I prefer to call them Global Narratives. What is true and what is pure speculation behind them? I did my homework! I researched them for you. But… Infodemic made that third chapter impossible by now. In a next book, may be. But I want to share with you what it would (will?) be about. This is the third chapter description I wrote:

I hope you, like me, do agree with Li Wenliang, the doctor who first advised a "SARS-like" disease was spreading in Wuhan, who said: "There should be more than one voice in a healthy society". There have always been many voices, and it is good and healthy there are, as long as society is wholeheartedly committed and able to fight ignorance and fear. The best way to fight ignorance and fear: knowledge. We will discuss the role played by Global Media and Social Networks. The irruption of fake news and censorship, the difference between a narrative and misinformation. And then, the funny part! We will check some global narratives and topics: Trade War and COVID-19, the apocalyptic Disease X, Big Pharma, Big Business, the infamous Super Spreaders, the prophetic Wuhan-400, the link between 5G and the Wuhan epidemic, the mysterious Wuhan Level-4 Laboratory: The Wuhan Institute of Virology, and the last but not the least, some dark speculations about Depopulation Methods and Bioweapons.

I will invite you to Choose your own adventure and finally I will share with you My Personal Narrative and some good, good, very good questions.

I would love to write all this for you.

One last word. You will see repeatedly along the book the titles **"Further recommended reading" or "Highly further recommended reading". Please DO NOT SKIP THEM!** I personally selected them for you among thousands of pages in the web. Some of them, mostly those quoted in Chapter Two, are essential.

I hope you find this book useful and enjoyable. Thank you so much.

CHAPTER ONE
What you need to Know

Words you need to know

Infectious disease

Infectious diseases, also called communicable diseases, are disorders caused by organisms — such as bacteria, viruses, fungi or parasites. Many organisms live in and on our bodies. They are normally harmless or even helpful. But under certain conditions, some organisms may cause disease. Some — but not all — infectious diseases can be passed from person to person. Infectious diseases that spread from person to person are said to be contagious. Infectious diseases that pass from animals to humans are called zoonotic diseases.

Contagious diseases (such as the flu, colds, or strep throat) spread from person to person in several ways. One way is through direct physical contact, like shaking hands, hugging, touching or kissing a person who has the infection. An infectious microbe also may travel through the air in tiny droplets expelled when someone nearby sneezes or coughs.

Sometimes people get contagious diseases by touching or using something an infected person has touched or used — like sharing a straw, touching a door knob, or stepping into the shower after someone who has athlete's foot. And sexually transmitted diseases (STDs) are spread through all types of sex — oral, anal, or vaginal.

However, infectious diseases are not the first global death causes. Causes of death vary significantly between countries: non-communicable diseases dominate in rich countries, whereas infectious diseases remain high at lower incomes. The world is making progress against infectious diseases. As a consequence, more people are dying from non-communicable diseases.

Virus

Virus are infectious agents like bacteria. But virus, unlike bacteria, are unable to reproduce by themselves.

A virus is a biological agent that reproduces inside the cells of living hosts. When infected by a virus, a host cell is forced to produce thousands of identical copies of the original virus at an extraordinary rate. Unlike most living things, viruses cannot reproduce by themselves; so new viruses are assembled in the infected host cell. But unlike still simpler infectious agents, viruses contain genes, which gives them the ability to mutate and evolve. Over 5,000 species of viruses have been discovered.

The origins of viruses are unclear: some may have evolved from plasmids—pieces of DNA that can move between cells—while others may have evolved from bacteria. A virus consists of two or three parts: genes, a protein coat and, only in some cases, an envelope made of fats. First: the genes, made from either DNA or RNA, are long molecules that carry genetic information; seconds, the protein coat that protects the genes; and third, in some viruses, an envelope of fat that surrounds the protein coat and is used, in combination with specific receptors, to enter a new host cell. Viruses vary in shape from the simple helical and icosahedral to more complex structures. Viruses range in size from 20 to 300 nanometers; it would take 33,000 to 500,000 of them, side by side, to stretch to 1 centimeter (0.39 in).

Viruses spread in many ways. Just as viruses are very specific as to which host species or tissue they attack, each species of virus relies on a particular method for propagation. Plant viruses are often spread from plant to plant by insects and other organisms, known as vectors. Some viruses of animals, including humans, are spread by exposure to infected bodily fluids. Viruses such as influenza are spread through the air by droplets when people cough or sneeze. Viruses such as norovirus are transmitted by the fecal–oral route, which involves the contamination of hands, food and water with feces. Rotavirus is often spread by direct contact with infected children. The human immunodeficiency virus, HIV, is transmitted by bodily fluids transferred during sex. Others, such as the Dengue virus, are spread by blood-sucking insects, like mosquitos, ticks and fleas, which are called the vectors of the disease.

Viral infections can cause disease in humans, animals and even plants. However, they are usually eliminated by the immune system, conferring lifetime immunity to the host for that virus. Antibiotics have no effect on viruses, but antiviral drugs have been developed to treat life-threatening viral infections. Most viral infections resolve spontaneously in immunocompetent individuals. The aim of antiviral therapy is to minimize symptoms and infectivity as well as to shorten the duration of illness. As viruses use the host cell to reproduce themselves, antiviral drugs are designed to affect the cells ability to reproduce. These drugs act by arresting the viral replication cycle at various stages. Because viruses are intracellular parasites, it is difficult to find drugs that interfere with viral replication without also harming the host cells. Unlike other antimicrobials, antiviral drugs do not deactivate or destroy the virus but act by inhibiting its replication. In this way, they prevent the viral load from increasing to a point where it could cause pathogenesis, allowing the body's innate immune mechanisms to neutralize the virus. Currently, antiviral therapy is available only for a limited number of infections. Most of the antiviral drugs currently available are used to treat infections caused by HIV, herpes viruses, hepatitis B and C viruses, and influenza A and B viruses.

Endemic, Epidemic and Pandemic diseases

All this three words include the element "dem" which comes from the ancient Greek word "demos", the same as in "democracy": demos, the people plus a preposition:

Epidemic: ancient Greek preposition "Epi", which means among, plus "demos": among the people;

Endemic: ancient Greek preposition "En", which means in, plus "demos": in the people;

Pandemic: ancient Greek preposition "pan", which means all, plus "demos": all the peoples.

So, an epidemic is a widespread occurrence of an infectious disease in a community at a particular time.

Endemic is an adjective that refers to a disease or condition regularly found among particular people or in a certain area.

A disease becomes pandemic when it spreads beyond a region to infect large numbers of people worldwide.

Please note that none of these words refers to the severity of an illness. They all refer to the disease's geographical or numerical extension at a given time. Endemics imply a question about a particular location. For example, a typical question about an endemic disease: where is malaria endemic?

Epidemics always imply a question about number, for example: how many seasonal flu cases are expected this year? and pandemics both questions, How many? and where? How many COVID-19 cases worldwide up today?

Ro or Basic Reproduction Number

In Epidemiology, the basic reproduction number (sometimes called basic reproductive ratio, and denoted R0, pronounced R naught or R zero) of an infection can be thought of as the expected number of cases directly generated by one case in a population where all individuals are susceptible to infection.

R0 is neither a biological constant for a pathogen nor a measure of disease severity. R0 is affected by many factors such as environmental conditions (such as temperature or humidity), and biological and sociobehavioral characteristics of the infected population (as like, for example, habits, hygiene). Furthermore, R0 values are usually estimated from mathematical models, not from empirical research. And so, this estimated values, as like as all estimated values, are dependent on the model used and are dependent also on the values of other parameters. R0 does not by itself alone give an estimate of how fast an infection spreads in the population.

So, what is the basic reproduction number or R0 used for? The most important uses of R0 are determining if an emerging infectious disease can spread in a population. In commonly used infection models, when R0 > 1 the infection will be able to start spreading in a population, because each infected individual will pass the pathogen to more than one person, so the number of infected people will get bigger over time This will not be the case if R0 < 1, in which case the number of infected persons will diminish over time. Generally, the larger the value of R0, the harder it is to control the epidemic.

The basic reproduction number is affected by several factors including the duration of infectivity of affected patients, the infectiousness of the pathogen, and the number of susceptible people in the population that the affected patients are in contact with.

Some Ro values of well know infectious diseases:

Measles 12-18

Influenza (1918 Strain) 2-3

AIDS and SARS 2-5

COVID-19 1.4-3.8

MERS 0.3-0.8

During an epidemic the infected persons will go through different stages, which are relevant to the spreading of the disease:

Exposed: an individual is infected, but has no symptoms and does not yet infect others. This is the first phase of Incubation Period.

Latent infectious: an individual is infected, has no symptoms, but does infect others. The duration of this latent infectious state is variable (both for different pathogens and for different patients) and difficult to determine. Generally speaking, the longer this phase, the bigger the potential of transmission, because the individual is able to infect others during this period and he himself is apparently healthy. This is the second phase of Incubation Period.

An individual is infected, has symptoms, and does infect others. During this period, it is extremely important how the infected person behaves: does he ask for help? Is the needed help available? Does he trust authorities or does he fear them? Will he be careful not to spread the disease? Does he have the knowledge and the material means (these material means could be as basic as some money, transportation, a phone, but some people may not have them) to do so?

Isolation after diagnosis: measures are taken to prevent further infections, for example by isolating the patient.

For example, SARS disease has a higher case fatality rate (around 10%, Influenza´s is less than 1%) and a higher Ro value than Influenza (2-5 and 2-3 respectively), but as SARS onset of symptoms is faster and more severe, and do require medical treatment, SARS is most usually diagnosed promptly. So, the patient is rapidly isolated and can no longer spread the disease. This is the reason why the number of deaths caused by the 1918 Spanish Flu outbreak was so terribly high (estimated between twenty and forty million worldwide), and the 2002 SARS outbreak caused (only) 774 deaths.

The same goes for Seasonal Flu, which causes between 300.000 and

650.000 deaths worldwide annually. And, apparently, this is the case for COVID-19 also. COVID-19 shows just mild, flu-like symptoms, for more than the 80% of patients.

The World Health Organization said that the novel coronavirus does not seem to be as "deadly as other coronaviruses including SARS and MERS" At a briefing on February 17th, WHO's director general, Tedros Adhanom Ghebreyesus, said that more than 80% of patients with covid-19 have a "mild disease and will recover" and that it is fatal in 2% of reported cases. In comparison, the 2003 outbreak of Severe Acute Respiratory Syndrome (SARS) had a case fatality rate of around 10% (8098 cases and 774 deaths), while Middle East Respiratory Syndrome (MERS) killed 34% of infected people between 2012 and 2019 (2494 cases and 858 deaths).

However, despite the lower case fatality rate, covid-19, as early as by February 17th, resulted in more deaths (1871) than SARS and MERS combined (1632).

Mortality Rate and Case Fatality Rate

And here we are, finally considering the most dreadful number: **Mortality Rate or Death Rate.**

The Crude Death Rate or Mortality Rate is the total number of deaths in a specified geographic area (country, state, county, etc.) divided by the total population for the same geographic area (for a specified time period, usually a calendar year) and multiplied by 100,000. Note that deaths are not classified according any criterion (cause of death, age, sex); the total number of deaths is divided by the total number of individuals in the group under study. But this is not what we all worry about now.

What we are really interested on now is what Epidemiologists call **Case Fatality Rate**, or **Case Fatality Ratio (CFR).** Case Fatality Rate is the proportion of people who die from a specified disease among all individuals diagnosed with the disease over a certain period of time. Or, simply put, total number of deaths caused by a disease divided by the total number of diagnosed cases for the same disease over a given period of time. Case fatality rate typically is used as a measure of disease severity and is often used for prognosis, and also to evaluate alternative treatments' relative efficacy. Case fatality rates are not constant; they can vary between populations, (different case fatality rates for different cultures, age or gender groups) and over time because Case Fatality Rates depend on the interplay between the causative agent of disease, the host, and the environment, as well as on the available treatments and the quality of patient care. For example, consider the Case Fatality Rate for bacterial diseases before and after antibiotics are available. The first antibiotics were prescribed in the late 1930s. From then on, bacterial infection, as a cause of death, plummeted. Between 1944 and 1972 human life expectancy jumped (UP!) by eight years. This eight years' increase (if you think, this is really a very remarkable increase, of over a 10 % in life expectancy) is largely credited to the introduction of antibiotics.

But, if you carefully consider the definition above, that is, "Case Fatality Rate is the proportion of people who die from a specified disease among all individuals diagnosed with the disease over a certain period of time", you will notice that to calculate the Case Fatality Rate we need two numbers: the total number of deaths effectively caused by the illness, and the total number of diagnosed cases of the illness during a given period of time. Sadly, those numbers are not easily determined during an epidemics outbreak.

Because, how could you diagnose a case of a novel disease? You don´t even have a name for it yet! And of course you neither have specific lab tests, nor a clinical description of the symptoms. You will have to learn as you go.

What you will surely have, during the first days, are severely ill patients, and dead patients. Later on you will be able to relate those patients and deaths to the novel disease. This is quite possibly one of the reasons why Case Fatality Rates tend to decrease as the epidemic develops, because the first registered cases are usually those that required medical treatment.

And this brings us to consider the other number we need to calculate the Case Fatality Rate: the total number of diagnosed cases. And this is highly related to the severity of the illness, among other factors.

If, let´s say, the 100% of patients of a given illness require hospitalization, you will hopefully have an accurate number of cases, because most patients will show up at medical institutions. That's mostly the case of the most severe human coronaviruses, SARS and MERS.

What would happen if only a 20% of infected persons feel bad enough to go to the doctor? And what about an illness that goes asymptomatic for a long period of time, or for a big proportion of the infected? How could you possibly account those individuals among your registered cases? So it is not easy at all to determine the total number of infected people. This seems to be the case with COVID-19. Chinese officials say over an 80% of registered cases show only mild symptoms. They, amazingly, even detected an 1,2 percent of asymptomatic patients. What nobody knows is how many more asymptomatic and mildly symptomatic undetected cases there are for each confirmed case.

Much to worry it is the estimation by some experts that there are of up to ten unregistered cases for each diagnosed one. "You can't find things you don't look for," says Lipsitch, the Harvard epidemiologist. "We estimated that even high surveillance countries were missing about half their imported cases." (High surveillance countries use temperature screening devices in airports, and many other containment measures, to detect infected travelers before they enter the country). He predicts that a global coronavirus pandemic is "likely" and that 40 to 70 percent of the world's population could be infected (though they won't all become sick).

The good news is that, if this were true, the Case Fatality Rate for COVID-19 would be much, much lower than initially thought. Because the bigger the number of real cases (registered or not) the smaller the real Case Fatality Rate becomes, because the number of deaths tends to be more accurately registered than the number of infected individuals.

In the case of flu-like illnesses, like COVID-19, in the absence of specific lab tests, when you can only diagnose upon clinical observation of symptoms, you might quite easily underestimate the number of cases by ascribing some COVID-19 cases to the flu or, vice versa, overestimate the COVID-19 case numbers by ascribing to COVID-19 some flu cases.

And regarding the number of deaths, sometimes it is not easy to ascribe a death to a specific agent. In the case of the flu, or flu-like illnesses, most patients die as a consequence of a secondary infection, like bacterial pneumonias. Do you ascribe the death to Influenza or to the secondary infection agent? For COVID-19 the situation is apparently quite similar. You should stablish some criteria, and maintain the same criteria over time.

Community spread

Community spread means spread of an illness for which the source of infection is unknown. Or, put in other words, an illness whose successive contagions you can no longer trace up to a known and registered case. This implies that multiple active chains of contagion are simultaneously spreading the disease. Not anymore a single chain of cases you can register link by link, and hopefully isolate, but more like a tree shape whose branches split once and again.

On February 24th, the Center for Disease Control and Prevention warned that it expects the novel coronavirus that has sparked outbreaks around the world to begin spreading at a community level in the United States, as a top official said. And that disruptions to daily life could be "severe."

"As we've seen from recent countries with community spread, when it has hit those countries, it has moved quite rapidly. We want to make sure the American public is prepared," Nancy Messonnier, director of CDC's National Center for Immunization and Respiratory Diseases, told reporters.

Recommended further reading:

A single coronavirus case exposes a bigger problem: The scope of undetected U.S. spread is unknown By Hellen Branswell https://www.statnews.com/2020/02/27/a-single-coronavirus-case-exposes-a-bigger-problem-the-scope-of-undetected-u-s-spread-is-unknown/

It's likely there are more coronavirus cases in the United States than the numbers show By Elizabeth Cohen, Senior Medical Correspondent.

https://edition.cnn.com/2020/02/28/health/coronavirus-uncounted-cases-community-spread/index.html

Facts you need to know
Statistics: Global Death Causes

Recommended further reading

https://www.who.int/news-room/fact-sheets/detail/the-top-10-causes-of-death

https://en.wikipedia.org/wiki/List_of_causes_of_death_by_rate

Causes of Death Hannah Ritchie and Max Roser (2020) Published online at OurWorldInData.org. Retrieved from: 'https://ourworldindata.org/causes-of-death'

To understand emerging new phenomena, we are always highly dependent on what we already know. The known facts do, so, provide us, at least, with a silhouette, a negative shape of the newly discovered facts.

So, this way, the context made of known interwoven facts contours the new and yet unknown.

We should start from here, then. What do we know, almost since day 1, about COVID-19? What we know is that COVID-19 is a viral, potentially lethal, and potentially pandemic, disease.

So, let's review our context. What do we already know about lethal viral pandemics? This sounds really, really bad…

So stop and relax! Just a little. Do not panic yet. Because infectious diseases (among which the most lethal viral pandemics are classified) are not the first global cause of death.

Infectious diseases are not, neither, the second global cause of death.

Nor the third.

Infectious diseases, also called "communicable diseases", come, globally, in the fourth place.

And for a developed country citizen like you, not even that. Infectious, communicable diseases like COVID-19 only arrive in the sixth place!

As the World Health Organization says in an article published in 2018 about data collected worldwide during 2016: "Non-communicable diseases (NCDs) caused 71% of deaths globally, ranging from 37% in low-income countries to 88% in high-income countries. All but one of the 10 leading causes of death in high-income countries were NCDs."

Simply said, 88% of deaths in high-income countries, almost nine out of ten (nine out of ten! Did you read that?) were caused by non-communicable diseases. So, which are those non-communicable diseases? Ordered from most deadly to least deadly:

First, ischemic heart disease;

Second, stroke;

Third, Alzheimer disease and other dementias;

Fourth, Cancer (Trachea, Bronchus and Lung cancers)

Fifth, Chronic obstructive pulmonary disease;

Seventh, Diabetes Mellitus;

Eighth, Road Injury

Ninth, Cancer (Liver)

Tenth, Cancer (Stomach)

The sixth place, I repeat, loudly, THE SIXTH place, is for lower respiratory infections. Such as pneumonia.

Note that, as the WHO says, all but one of the 10 leading causes of death in high-income countries were NCDs, or vice versa, only one among the ten leading causes of death in high-income countries is a communicable or infectious disease.

In this excellent article from https://ourworldindata.org from the University of Oxford, written by Hannah Ritchie and Max Roser (2020) - "Causes of Death". Published online at OurWorldInData.org. Retrieved from: 'https://ourworldindata.org/causes-of-death' [Online Resource] you will find the following

"Summary:

Cardiovascular diseases are the leading cause of death globally.

The second biggest cause are cancers.

Causes of death vary significantly between countries: non-communicable diseases dominate in rich countries, whereas infectious diseases remain high at lower incomes.

The world is making progress against infectious diseases. As a consequence, more people are dying from non-communicable diseases.

Fewer people die at a young age. Almost half of all people who die are 70 years and older.

Leading risk factors for premature death globally include high blood pressure, smoking, obesity, high blood sugar and environmental risk factors including air pollution.

There is a large difference between what people die from and which causes of death receive news coverage."

It seems so that we should worry much more about, and I loudly repeat, we should worry much more about The Leading Risk Factors for Premature Death, which globally include High Blood Pressure, Smoking, Obesity, High Blood Sugar and environmental risk factors including air pollution.

These should be our most dreaded pandemics. Because they are. They really are. But, and there is always a "but", they are not, at least, we do not perceive them as the lethal pandemics they indeed are. Because, as this great article (Read complete article here: Hannah Ritchie and Max Roser (2020) - "Causes of Death". Published online at OurWorldInData.org. Retrieved from: 'https://ourworldindata.org/causes-of-death') also says, "There is a large difference between what people die from and which causes of death receive news coverage". I repeat. Again. Loudly:

There is a large difference between what people die from and which causes of death receive news coverage.

And talking about causes of death which receive news coverage. Let´s talk about Viral Pandemics.

Viral Pandemics

Recommended further reading: Everything you need to know about pandemics by Yvette Brazier,

A pandemic is usually caused by a new virus strain or subtype that becomes easily transmissible between humans, or by bacteria that become resistant to antibiotic treatment.

Humans may have little or no immunity against a new virus.

In the case of seasonal influenza outbreaks, or epidemics, are generally caused by subtypes of a virus that is already circulating among people. So part of the population may have already developed a certain immunity against the virus.

Pandemics, on the other hand, are generally caused by novel subtypes. These subtypes have not circulated among people before. And this is the reason why the population may have little or no immunity for this new virus.

This is also why a pandemic affect more people and can be more deadly than an epidemic.

After the pandemic emerges and spreads, humans develop some immunity. And like a wave, the pandemic peaks, stabilizes and then fades. Then, the virus subtype can circulate among humans for several years, causing occasional outbreaks.

Many institutions around the world, like the World Health Organization (WHO) and the Centers for Disease Control and Prevention (CDC) of different countries, monitor the behavior and movements of the virus.

History

The Spanish flu pandemic, from 1918 to 1920, is supposed to have caused, according to different authors, from 20 million and up to 100 million lives. It is considered the worst in history. The Black Death claimed the lives of over 75 million people in the 14th Century (about 30 to 60 % of the European population at the time).

Some pandemics and epidemics:

Black Death 1346-1350
Cholera 1899-1923

Spanish flu (H1N1) 1918-1920

Asian flu (H2N2) 1957-1958

Hong Kong flu 1968-1969

SARS 2002

Avian flu (H1N1) 2009

MERS 2012

The WHO divided the development of an Influenza pandemic in six stages. As Influenza is a viral disease, we will apply this description to other viral pandemics:

Stage 1

No animal influenza virus circulating among animals has been reported to cause infection in humans.

Stage 2

An animal influenza virus circulating in domesticated or wild animals is known to have caused infection in humans and is therefore considered a specific potential pandemic threat.

Stage 3

An animal or human-animal influenza reassortant virus has caused sporadic cases or small clusters of disease in people, but it has not resulted in human-to-human transmission sufficient to sustain community-level outbreaks.

Stage 4

Human-to-human transmission of an animal or human-animal influenza reassortant virus able to sustain community-level outbreaks has been verified.

Stage 5

The same identified virus has caused sustained community level outbreaks in two or more countries in one WHO region.

Phase 6

In addition to the criteria defined in Phase 5, the same virus has caused sustained community level outbreaks in at least one other country in another

WHO region.

This description of a pandemic´s development was not yet applied to the COVID-19 disease, as the World Health Organization has refused to apply the name pandemic to the disease.

The WHO also describes two important periods following the pandemic spread

Post-peak period

Levels of pandemic influenza in most countries with adequate surveillance have dropped below peak levels.

Post-pandemic period

Levels of influenza activity have returned to the levels seen for seasonal influenza in most countries with adequate surveillance.

Modern pandemics

If an influenza pandemic were to emerge today, the following problems could arise:

People today are more international mobile and more likely to live in cities than in the past, factors which increase the risk of a virus spreading.

Faster communication increases the risk of panic, and the chance that people who may be infected will travel in an attempt to escape the disease, potentially taking the virus with them.

It can take months or years for a vaccine to become available, because pandemic viruses are novel agents.

Medical facilities would be overwhelmed, and there could be shortages of personnel to provide vital community services, due to both the demand and illness.

Concerns

Pandemics involve novel agents; because of this, medical science must keep on its toes.

Medical science has advanced rapidly in recent years, but it is unlikely ever to offer full protection from a possible pandemic, because of the novel nature of the diseases involved.

Spanish Flu
The worst-case scenario for pandemic planning

Recommended further reading:

Lessons from a Century After the Flu Epidemic of 1918: How Conventional Medicine Killed Millions and How Homeopathic Medicines Saved Millions

https://articles.mercola.com/sites/articles/archive/2018/12/06/homeopathic-remedies-for-influenza.aspx

Transmissibility of 1918 pandemic influenza by Mills, C., Robins, J. & Lipsitch https://www.nature.com/articles/nature03063

In the article Transmissibility of 1918 pandemic influenza, the authors say (see reference above): "The 1918 influenza pandemic killed 20–40 million people worldwide, and is seen as a worst-case scenario for pandemic planning. Like other pandemic influenza strains, the 1918 A/H1N1 strain spread extremely rapidly. A measure of transmissibility and of the stringency of control measures required to stop an epidemic is the reproductive number, which is the number of secondary cases produced by each primary case. Here we obtained an estimate of the reproductive number for 1918 influenza… from 45 US cities: the median value is less than three… These results strongly suggest that the reproductive number for 1918 pandemic influenza is not large relative to many other infectious diseases. In theory, a similar novel influenza subtype could be controlled. But because influenza is frequently transmitted before a specific diagnosis is possible… aggressive transmission reducing measures will probably be required."

It was thought that the Spanish Flu would have had a very high transmission rate, like measles, for example. One measles infected patient is expected to transmit the disease to average 16 to 18 other persons. But studies stablished a relatively low transmission rate, with a medium value less than three. Such transmission values are generally thought as containable. But, how did the Spanish Flu spread worldwide as it did? It spread worldwide as it did because "influenza is frequently transmitted before a specific diagnosis is possible". And this is, sadly, the case with COVID-19.

This is one of the reasons why several studies indicate border screenings with temperature scanners are not effective. "I think airport scanning is more of a political measure than a practical measure. It might calm people down and demonstrate that the government is doing something, but as for public health, it's not very useful," says Coker, an emeritus public health professor. These screenings must catch people in a very narrow window, during a more or less short time when they are well enough to travel, but sick enough to detect. Temperature scanners will not find anyone whose fever may have subsided after a Tylenol on the plane. And simply because someone doesn't present clinical symptoms, it doesn't mean they aren't sick. Asymptomatic patients still in the incubation phase have spread coronavirus, according to doctors.

And we know the epidemic in China almost doubled the number of cases each week. This is coincidental with a transmission rate estimated of 2.2, if, and only if, asymptomatic patients are able to spread the disease.

So it seems we are (relatively) fortunate because an illness with a transmission ability comparable to the Spanish Flu is causing so (relatively) little number of deaths.

Coronaviruses

Recommended further reading:

Coronavirus Infections—More Than Just the Common Cold by Catharine I. Paules, MD; Hilary D. Marston, MD, MPH; Anthony S. Fauci, MD

https://jamanetwork.com/journals/jama/fullarticle/2759815

Article Information: Corresponding Author: Anthony S. Fauci, MD, Laboratory of Immunoregulation, National Institute of Allergy and Infectious Diseases, 31 Center Dr, MSC 2520, Bldg 31, Room 7A-03, Bethesda, MD 20892-2520 (afauci@niaid.nih.gov). Published Online: January 23, 2020. doi:10.1001/jama.2020.0757

Please note that all the info below was collected from the most reliable sources, mostly from the World Health Organization and Centers for Disease Control and Prevention of the United States online sites and public communications. In the section **Surfing the World Wide Web** we will discuss some trending topics on the Web, news, data analysis and forecasts.

Coronaviruses (CoV) are a large family of viruses. Coronaviruses are named for the crown-like spikes on their surface. There are four main sub-groupings of coronaviruses, known as alpha, beta, gamma, and delta.

Several known coronaviruses are circulating in animals that have not yet infected humans.

Sometimes coronaviruses that infect animals can evolve and make people sick and so become a new human coronavirus.

These Coronaviruses are called zoonotic, because they are transmitted between animals and people. Three recent examples of this are 2019-nCoV, SARS-CoV, and MERS-CoV.

According to the WHO, detailed investigations found that SARS-CoV was transmitted from civet cats to humans and MERS-CoV from dromedary camels to humans.

Human Coronavirus Types

Human coronaviruses were first identified in the mid-1960s. The seven known coronaviruses that can infect people are:

1-**229E** (alpha coronavirus)

2-**NL63** (alpha coronavirus)

3-**OC43** (beta coronavirus)

4-**HKU1** (beta coronavirus)

5-**MERS-CoV** (the beta coronavirus that causes Middle East Respiratory Syndrome, or MERS)

6-**SARS-CoV** (the beta coronavirus that causes severe acute respiratory syndrome, or SARS)

7-**SARS-CoV-2** (the novel coronavirus that causes coronavirus disease 2019, or COVID-19)

At CDC site (https://www.cdc.gov/coronavirus/general-information.html) you can find this great info about Human Coronaviruses. I have summarized it for you.

1 to 4 Common Human Coronaviruses aka Common Cold

People around the world commonly get infected with human coronaviruses 229E, NL63, OC43, and HKU1.

Common human coronaviruses, including types 229E, NL63, OC43, and HKU1, usually cause mild to moderate upper-respiratory tract illnesses, like the common cold. Most people get infected with one or more of these viruses at some point in their lives. Please note that this information applies to common human coronaviruses and should not be confused with Coronavirus Disease-2019 (formerly referred to as 2019 Novel Coronavirus).

Symptoms of common human coronaviruses (also known as common cold)

- runny nose
- sore throat
- headache
- fever
- cough
- general feeling of being unwell

Human coronaviruses can sometimes cause lower respiratory tract illnesses, such as pneumonia or bronchitis. This is more common in people with cardiopulmonary disease, people with weakened immune systems, infants, and older adults.

Transmission of common human coronaviruses (also known as common cold)

Common human coronaviruses usually spread from an infected person to others through

- the air by coughing and sneezing
- close personal contact, like touching or shaking hands
- touching an object or surface with the virus on it, then touching your mouth, nose, or eyes before washing your hands

In the United States, people usually get infected with common human coronaviruses in the fall and winter, but you can get infected at any time of the year. Young children are most likely to get infected, but people can have multiple infections in their lifetime.

Preventing viral respiratory infections

Protect yourself from getting sick

- wash your hands often with soap and water for at least 20 seconds
- avoid touching your eyes, nose, or mouth with unwashed hands
- avoid close contact with people who are sick

Protect others when you are sick

- stay home while you are sick
- avoid close contact with others
- cover your mouth and nose when coughing or sneezing
- clean and disinfect objects and surfaces

Treatment for common human coronaviruses

There is no vaccine to protect you against human coronaviruses and there are no specific treatments for illnesses caused by human coronaviruses. Most people with common human coronavirus illness will recover on their own. However, to relieve your symptoms you can:

- take pain and fever medications (Caution: do not give aspirin to children. It might cause severe complications)
- use a room humidifier or take a hot shower to help ease a sore throat and cough
- drink plenty of liquids
- stay home and rest

If you are concerned about your symptoms, contact your healthcare provider.

Testing for common human coronaviruses

Sometimes, respiratory secretions are tested to figure out which specific germ is causing your symptoms.

- If you are found to be infected with a common coronavirus (229E, NL63, OC43, and HKU1), that does not mean you are infected with the 2019 novel coronavirus.

• There are different tests to determine if you are infected with 2019 novel coronavirus. Your

healthcare provider can determine if you should be tested. You can find the full text here: https://www.cdc.gov/coronavirus/types.html

5-MERS- CoV

(the beta coronavirus that causes Middle East Respiratory Syndrome, or MERS)

MERS is the acronym for Middle East Respiratory Syndrome.

The Middle East Respiratory Syndrome is a severe acute respiratory illness caused by the MERS-CoV coronavirus.

MERS-CoV infection was first reported in September 2012 in Saudi Arabia, but an outbreak in April 2012 in Jordan was confirmed retrospectively. As of 2018, worldwide, more than two thousand cases of MERS-CoV infection (with at least 750 related deaths, which means above a 33% case fatality rate) have been reported from twenty-seven countries around the globe; all cases of MERS have been linked through travel to or residence in countries in and near the Arabian Peninsula, with more than 80% in Saudi Arabia. The largest known outbreak of MERS outside the Arabian Peninsula occurred in the Republic of Korea in 2015. The outbreak was associated with a traveler returning from the Arabian Peninsula. Cases have also been confirmed in France, Germany, Italy, Tunisia, and the United Kingdom in patients who were either transferred there for care or became ill after returning from the Middle East.

Preliminary seroprevalence studies indicate that the infection is not widespread in Saudi Arabia.

The WHO considers the risk of contracting MERS-CoV infection to be very low for pilgrims traveling to Saudi Arabia for Umrah and Hajj; last year's (2018) Hajj did not result in an increase of patients with MERS-CoV infection. For additional information concerning risks of contracting MERS for pilgrims traveling to Saudi Arabia for Umrah and Hajj please visit World Health Organization interim travel advice on MERS-CoV for pilgrimages to the Kingdom of Saudi Arabia https://www.who.int/ith/updates/20130725/en/

Demographics of MERS

Median age of patients with MERS-CoV is 56 years old, and the male:female ratio is about 1.6:1. Infection tends to be more severe in elderly patients and in patients with a preexisting disorder such as diabetes, a chronic heart disorder, or a chronic renal disorder.

Transmission of MERS-CoV

MERS-CoV may be transmitted from person to person via direct contact, respiratory droplets, or aerosols. Person-to-person transmission has been established by the development of infection in people whose only risk was close contact with people who had MERS.

The reservoir of MERS-CoV is thought to be dromedary camels, but the mechanism of transmission from camels to humans is unknown. Most reported cases involved direct human-to-human transmission in health care settings. If MERS is suspected in a patient, infection control measures must be initiated promptly to prevent transmission in health care settings.

Symptoms and Signs

The incubation period for MERS-CoV is about 5 days.

Most reported cases have involved severe respiratory illness requiring hospitalization, with a case fatality rate of about 35%; however, at least 21% of patients had mild or no symptoms. Fever, chills, myalgia, and cough are common. GI symptoms (e.g., diarrhea, vomiting, abdominal pain) occur in about one third of patients. Manifestations may be severe enough to require treatment in an ICU, but recently, the proportion of such cases has declined sharply.

Diagnosis

Real-time reverse-transcriptase PCR (RT-PCR) testing of upper and lower respiratory secretions and serum

MERS should be suspected in patients who have an unexplained acute febrile lower respiratory infection and who have had either of the following within 14 days of symptom onset:

Travel to or residence in an area where MERS has recently been reported or where transmission could have occurred

Contact with a health care facility where MERS has been transmitted

Close contact with a patient who was ill with suspected MERS

MERS should also be suspected in patients who have had close contact with a patient with suspected MERS and who have a fever whether they have respiratory symptoms or not.

In all patients, chest imaging detects abnormalities, which may be subtle or extensive, unilateral or bilateral. In some patients, levels of LDH and AST are elevated and/or levels of platelets and lymphocytes are low. A few patients have acute kidney injury. Disseminated intravascular coagulation and hemolysis may develop.

Treatment

Treatment of MERS is supportive. To help prevent spread from suspected cases, health care practitioners should use standard, contact, and airborne precautions.

There is no vaccine, nor specific medication available for this disease yet.

6-SARS-CoV

(the beta coronavirus that causes severe acute respiratory syndrome, or SARS)

SARS is the acronym for Severe Acute Respiratory Syndrome. SARS is a viral respiratory illness caused by a coronavirus called SARS-associated coronavirus (SARS-CoV). SARS is much more severe than other coronavirus infections. SARS is an influenza-like illness that occasionally leads to progressively severe respiratory insufficiency.

SARS-CoV was first detected in the Guangdong province of China in November 2002 and subsequently spread to more than thirty countries in North America, South America, Europe, and Asia before the SARS global outbreak was contained. In this outbreak, more than eight thousand cases were reported worldwide, with 774 deaths (about a 10% case fatality rate). The SARS-CoV outbreak was the first time that the CDC advised against travel to a region. This outbreak subsided, and no new cases have been identified since 2004. The immediate source was presumed to be civet cats, which had been infected through contact with a bat before they were sold in a live meat market. Bats are frequent carrier hosts of coronaviruses.

Transmission of SARS

SARS-CoV is transmitted from person to person by close personal contact. It is thought to be transmitted most readily by respiratory droplets produced when an infected person coughs or sneezes.

Diagnosis of SARS is made clinically, and treatment is supportive. There are no specific vaccines nor specific medications for this disease. Coordination of prompt and rigid infection control practices helped control the 2002 outbreak rapidly.

Since 2004, there have not been any known cases of SARS reported anywhere in the world.

7- SARS-CoV-2

On February 11, 2020 the World Health Organization announced an official name for the disease that is causing the 2019 novel coronavirus outbreak, first identified in Wuhan China. The new name of this disease is coronavirus disease 2019, abbreviated as COVID-19. In COVID-19, 'CO' stands for 'corona,' 'VI' for 'virus,' and 'D' for disease. Formerly, this disease was referred to as "2019 novel coronavirus" or "2019-nCoV."

There are many types of human coronaviruses including some that commonly cause mild upper-respiratory tract illnesses. COVID-19 is a new disease, caused be a novel (or new) coronavirus that has not previously been seen in humans. However, the new coronavirus' genetic sequence is 79.5% similar to SARS, the coronavirus that killed hundreds and devastated local economies in 2003.

Transmission of SARS-CoV-2

Current understanding about how the virus that causes coronavirus disease 2019 (COVID-19) spreads is largely based on what is known about similar coronaviruses.

The virus is thought to spread mainly from person-to-person.

Between people who are in close contact with one another (within about 6 feet)

Via respiratory droplets produced when an infected person coughs or sneezes.

These droplets can land in the mouths or noses of people who are nearby or possibly be inhaled into the lungs.

Spread from contact with infected surfaces or objects

It may be possible that a person can get COVID-19 by touching a surface or object that has the virus on it and then touching their own mouth, nose, or possibly their eyes, but this is not thought to be the main way the virus spreads.

When does spread happen?

People are thought to be most contagious when they are most symptomatic (the sickest).

Some spread might be possible before people show symptoms; there have been reports of this with this new coronavirus, but this is not thought to be the main way the virus spreads.

How efficiently does the virus spread?

How easily a virus spreads from person-to-person can vary. Some viruses are highly contagious (like measles), while other viruses are less so. Another factor is whether the spread continues over multiple generations of people (if spread is sustained). The virus that causes COVID-19 seems to be spreading easily and sustainably in Hubei province and other parts of China. In the United States, spread from person-to-person has occurred only among a few close contacts and has not spread any further to date.

Symptoms and signs

For confirmed coronavirus disease 2019 (COVID-19) cases, reported illnesses have ranged from mild symptoms to severe illness and death. Symptoms can include:

Fever

Cough

Shortness of breath

Symptoms of COVID-19 may appear in as few as 2 days or as long as 14 days after exposure. This is based on what has been seen previously as the incubation period of MERS-CoV viruses.

Treatment

Treatment of COVID-19 is supportive.

There is no vaccine, nor specific medication available for this disease yet.

COVID-19 Case Fatality Rate

The paper conclusions are the following: (Find full text here http://weekly.chinacdc.cn/en/article/id/e53946e2-c6c4-41e9-9a9b-fea8db1a8f51)

"Results

Patients

A total of 72,314 unique records were extracted and data from all records were included in the analysis. Thus, all 72,314 individuals diagnosed with COVID-19 as of February 11, 2020, were included in the analysis. Among them, 44,672 cases (61.8%) were confirmed, 16,186 cases (22.4%) were suspected, 10,567 cases (14.6%) were clinically diagnosed, and 889 cases (1.2%) were asymptomatic.

Baseline characteristics of confirmed cases (n=44,672) are presented in Table 1. A majority were aged 30–69 years (77.8%), male (51.4%), farmers or laborers (22.0%), and diagnosed in Hubei Province (74.7%). Most patients reported Wuhan-related exposures (85.8%) and were classified as mild cases (80.9%).

Deaths, Case Fatality Rates, and Mortality

As shown in Table 1, a total of 1,023 deaths have occurred among 44,672 confirmed cases for an overall case fatality rate of 2.3%. Additionally, these 1,023 deaths occurred during 661,609 PD of observed time, for a mortality rate of 0.015/10 PD.

The ≥80 age group had the highest case fatality rate of all age groups at 14.8%. Case fatality rate for males was 2.8% and for females was 1.7%. By occupation, patients who reported being retirees had the highest case fatality rate at 5.1%, and patients in Hubei Province had a >7-fold higher case fatality rate at 2.9% compared to patients in other provinces (0.4%). While patients who reported no comorbid conditions had a case fatality rate of 0.9%, patients with comorbid conditions had much higher rates—10.5% for those with cardiovascular disease, 7.3% for diabetes, 6.3% for chronic respiratory disease, 6.0% for hypertension, and 5.6% for cancer. Case fatality rate was also very high for cases categorized as critical at 49.0%.

Age Distribution and Sex Ratio

The age distribution of cases in Wuhan only, in Hubei Province overall, and in China overall are presented in Figure 1. The proportion of confirmed cases 30–79 years of age at baseline (i.e., date of diagnosis) was 89.8% for cases in Wuhan city versus 88.6% in Hubei overall (which includes Wuhan) and 86.6% in China overall (which includes Hubei Province and all 30 other provincial-level administrative divisions, or PLADs). The male-to-female ratio was 0.99:1 in Wuhan, 1.04:1 in Hubei, and 1.06:1 in China overall."

So: Almost 90% of confirmed cases were individuals from 30 to 79 years old. And very few confirmed cases among children aged 9 and younger (only 416), just about 1% of the total cases. None of them died.

Confirmed cases among children and teens aged 9 to 19 were very uncommon too; only 549 cases in that group, as little as 1.2%. There was a single death in that age group. On the other side of the spectrum, almost 15% of the people 80 years old and older, died.

It is difficult to tell if the low infection rates among children and teens means that kids actually don´t get infected, or if they get infected but rarely develop the disease and so go undetected. It seems that they do get infected but remain asymptomatic. Should we ask ourselves if they, anyway, are able to spread the disease. And it is quite possible that they do. Many experts think children are probably playing a role in spreading the virus. "If they are infected, there is no reason to believe that they will not transmit," experts say.

Recommended Further reading:

Time to use the p-word? Coronavirus enters dangerous new phase as outbreaks surge worldwide, scientists fear that COVID-19 might soon become pandemic. By Ellen Callaway https://www.nature.com/articles/d41586-020-00551-1

https://www.worldometers.info/coronavirus/coronavirus-expert-opinions/

Surfing the World Wide Web

"In its early stages, the epidemic doubled in size every 7.4 days. With a mean serial interval of 7.5 days (95% CI, 5.3 to 19), the basic reproductive number was estimated to be 2.2 (95% CI, 1.4 to 3.9).

On the basis of this information, there is evidence that human-to-human transmission has occurred among close contacts since the middle of December 2019. Considerable efforts to reduce transmission will be required to control outbreaks if similar dynamics apply elsewhere. Measures to prevent or reduce transmission should be implemented in populations at risk." (Quoted from the paper Early Transmission Dynamics in Wuhan, China, of Novel Coronavirus–Infected Pneumonia - Qun Li et al., New England Journal of Medicine, Jan. 29, 2020)

In the sections above we have studied the information provided by the most reliable sources, the World Health Organization and the Center for Disease Control of the United States.

But there is much more to learn around the web.

I have researched the web and in this section I will share with you the best, most useful info I found.

Info changes all the time, and develops all the time. The WHO officials talked about an infodemic going on. I must confess: I am infected. Infodemic, just as COVID-19, grows exponentially.

This is what I selected for you. Some hot topics discussed everywhere on the web like: COVID-19 and Influenza; COVID-19 Case fatality rate (CFR), COVID-19 Incubation Period and transmission, and COVID.19 and pets.

COVID-19 and Influenza

Recommended further reading:

https://jamanetwork.com/journals/jama/fullarticle/2762386

Much is said about COVID-19 and the flu. But numbers are crystal clear. Take a look:

Winter 2019-2020 Seasonal flu epidemic in the United States is considered moderately severe. But its numbers are impressive:

At least 29,000,000 ill patients

Above 13,000,000 physician visits

More than 280,000 hospitalizations

At least 16,000 deaths

105 pediatric influenza related deaths reported to the CDC

The United States population is 329.450.000 approximately. So almost a 9% of total population was ill during this winter only (data included cases registered before 2020, February 24th)

COVID-19 Case fatality rate (CFR)

"A consensus is needed on how to define and measure the seriousness of infection before the next pandemic"

Said Jessica Y. Wong, Heath Kelly, Dennis K. M. Ip, Joseph T. Wu, Gabriel M. Leung, and Benjamin J. Cowling in their 2013 paper Discussion of Case Fatality Rate for 2009 H1N1 epidemics

Recommended further reading:

https://www.worldometers.info/coronavirus/coronavirus-death-rate/

https://www.nytimes.com/2020/03/05/health/coronavirus-deaths-rates.html

https://www.medicalnewstoday.com/articles/why-are-covid-19-death-rates-so-hard-to-calculate-experts-weigh-in

https://edition.cnn.com/2020/02/21/health/coronavirus-reported-cases-covid-19-change-intl/index.html About How China changed the method for counting cases (only laboratory confirmed vs laboratory confirmed plus clinically diagnosed)

https://www.axios.com/coronavirus-at-brink-of-global-pandemic-5342192f-a486-41e3-acab-fe541a353e1b.html

https://www.theguardian.com/science/2020/jan/26/coronavirus-could-infect-100000-globally-experts-warn)

https://www.ncbi.nlm.nih.gov/pmc/articles/PMC3809029/Case fatality risk of influenza A(H1N1pdm09): a systematic review by Jessica Y. Wong, Heath Kelly,2,3 Dennis K. M. Ip, Joseph T. Wu, Gabriel M. Leung, and Benjamin J. Cowling Discussion of Case Fatality Rate for 2009 H1N1 epidemics.

In the paper "Case Fatality Risk of Influenza A (H1N1)" written as early as 2013, the authors conclude: "Our review highlights the difficulty in estimating the seriousness of infection with a novel influenza virus using the case fatality risk. In addition, substantial variability in age-specific estimates complicates the interpretation of the overall case fatality risk and comparisons among populations. A consensus is needed on how to define and measure the seriousness of infection before the next pandemic".

Live on TV President Trump said:

"I think the 3.4% is really a false number," he told Sean Hannity, one of his favorite conservative Fox News hosts, in a phone interview broadcast live.

"Now, this is just my hunch," Trump began, before continuing that "based on a lot of conversations with a lot of people that do this, because a lot of people will have this, and it's very mild – they'll get better very rapidly, they don't even see a doctor, they don't even call a doctor."

He went on: "You never hear about those people, so you can't put them down in the category of the overall population, in terms of this corona flu, and/or virus. So you just can't do that."

So, what are the facts? And why is this number, the Case Fatality rate so elusive?

The paper by the Chinese CDC quoted above, published in the Chinese Journal of Epidemiology, including more than 44,000 confirmed cases of Covid-19 in China as of February 11th, concludes that 80.9% of infections are classified as mild, 13.8% as severe and only 4.7% as critical. The number of deaths among those infected, known as the Fatality Rate, remains low but rises among those over 80 years old. The findings put the overall death rate of the Covid-19 virus at 2.3%.

A careful analysis of data shows that the Case Fatality Rate is calculated taking into account only the confirmed cases, not the grand total of cases considered in the study. The confirmed cases amount (only) up to 44.972 individuals over the 72.314 individuals diagnosed of COVID-19 included in the paper. The confirmed cases represent (only) the 61% of the grand total. I quote: "A total of 72,314 unique records were extracted and data from all records were included in the analysis. Thus, all 72,314 individuals diagnosed with COVID-19 as of February 11, 2020, were included in the analysis. Among them, 44,672 cases (61.8%) were confirmed, 16,186 cases (22.4%) were suspected, 10,567 cases (14.6%) were clinically diagnosed, and 889 cases (1.2%) were asymptomatic."

So if you consider confirmed cases plus clinically diagnosed cases, your universe sums up to 55.239 individuals. And the Case Fatality Rate would be 1,85 %.

If you consider, then, all 72.314 cases diagnosed, the Case Fatality Rate would be only 1,41%.

I understand that confirmed cases surely are the most relevant, but what about the rest? Those were also COVID-19 diagnoses.

Another curious detail: 1,2% (889 cases) appear both as asymptomatic and not among the confirmed cases. So they were not diagnosed clinically (because they were asymptomatic) and they were not confirmed by tests. So how where they diagnosed as COVID-19 patients? Anyways, we should add this 1,2% to the 80,9% of mild cases, as this 80,9% was calculated over the registered cases only. So the asymptomatic (who strangely enough showed up at the hospital) plus the mild cases total 82,1% of the individuals diagnosed for COVID-19. I should ask how many asymptomatic but infected individuals never showed up at the Hospital for each one who actually did? And how many mild cases were never reported? If you think about this, the real Case Fatality Rate falls and falls. And keeps falling… "We're going to see a diminution in the overall death rate. There's another whole cohort that is either asymptomatic or minimally symptomatic," Anthony Fauci, the director of the US National Institute of Allergy and Infectious Diseases said in February.

Neil Ferguson, a public health expert at Imperial College in the UK, said his "best guess" was that there were 100,000 affected by the virus even though there were only 2,000 confirmed cases at the time. That is, fifty cases remained undetected for each diagnosed one, (Read full article here: https://www.theguardian.com/science/2020/jan/26/coronavirus-could-infect-100000-globally-experts-warn)

Without going that far, the possibility of a significant number of unreported cases in the initial stages of the crisis should be taken into account when trying to calculate the Case Fatality Rate.

But the World Health Organization is rising controversy. At a briefing on February 17th, WHO's director general, Tedros Adhanom Ghebreyesus, said that more than 80% of patients with covid-19 have a "mild disease and will recover" and that it is fatal in 2% of reported cases. But on march 3rd he himself said that "Globally, about 3.4% of reported COVID-19 cases have died. By comparison, seasonal flu generally kills far fewer than 1% of those infected". (Read complete briefing here: https://www.who.int/dg/speeches/detail/who-director-general-s-opening-remarks-at-the-media-briefing-on-covid-19---3-march-2020)

The Case Fatality Rate as of Feb. 20 in China, according to the Report of the WHO-China Joint Mission published on February 28th are the following:

The Report of the WHO-China Joint Mission is based on 55,924 laboratory confirmed cases. Here are its findings on Case Fatality Ratio, or CFR:

"As of 20 February, 2,114 of the 55,924 laboratory confirmed cases have died (crude fatality ratio [CFR: 3.8%)

The overall CFR varies by location and intensity of transmission (i.e. 5.8% in Wuhan vs. 0.7% in other areas in China).

In China, the overall CFR was higher in the early stages of the outbreak (17.3% for cases with symptom onset from 1-10 January) and has reduced over time to 0.7% for patients with symptom onset after 1 February.

The Joint Mission noted that the standard of care has evolved over the course of the outbreak."

Again we are talking here about laboratory confirmed cases. Only laboratory confirmed cases are included. How many cases where only clinically diagnosed? And how many cases remained undetected? We don't know.

What we do know is COVID-19 Case Fatality Rate for other countries. Japan, for example. Japan reported 350 domestic cases and 6 deaths by march, 5th. That is a 1.7%. If you consider also Diamond Princess cases also, which are not included among the domestic cases reported, the CFR for Japan is even lower: 1.2% (almost a thousand cases and twelve deaths). You can check this information at the site of Japanese government (here: https://www.mhlw.go.jp/stf/seisakunitsuite/bunya/newpage_00032.html) According to official government reports from other counties, as of 12:00, Mar. 5, 93,866 infectious cases and 3,269 deaths were confirmed. (CFR 3.4%) These are some relevant data from this report, in numbers country by country:

China	80,409 cases	3,012 deaths	CFR 3.7%
South Korea	5,766 cases	35 deaths	CFR 0.6%
Iran	2,922 cases	92 deaths	CFR 3.4%
Italy	2,706 cases	107 deaths	CFR 3.9%
France	285 cases	4 deaths	CFR 1.4%
Spain	198 cases	1 deaths	CFR 0.5%
United States	129 cases	9 deaths	CFR 6.9%
Hong Kong	104 cases	2 deaths	CFR 1.9%
Australia	52 cases	2 deaths	CFR 1.8%
Thailand	43 cases	1 death	CFR 2.3 %
Taiwan	42 cases	1 death	CFR 2.3%
Iraq	32 cases	1 death	CFR 3.1%

Please note that the Case Fatality Rates are surprisingly variable among countries, ranging from 6.9% (United States) to 0.5% (Spain).

Among the four countries with more cases detected (China, South Korea, Iran and Italy) three out of four report Case Fatality Rates above 3.4%. South Korea only 0.6%.

Among all, two countries outstand: Korea, with this so low Case Fatality Rate of 0.6%, and de United States with the highest Case Fatality Rate: 6.9%. Italy is the second worse, with 3.9%. Why is South Korea rate so good? And why is the United States so bad? I would really like to know.

And the countries that reported confirmed cases of COVID-19 but no deaths are: Germany, 262 cases; Singapore, 112 cases; United Kingdom, 86; Switzerland, 58; Kuwait, 56; Bahrain, 51; Kingdom of the Netherlands,38; Sweden,35; Canada, 33; Norway, 33;   India, 29; Austria, 29; United Arab Emirates, 27; Iceland,   26; and Belgium,   23.

Again, why Germany and Singapore did not have any deaths considering the relatively high number of cases? What did they do differently?

Why 3.4% is likely an overestimate

(Read full article in:https://www.medicalnewstoday.com/articles/why-are-covid-19-death-rates-so-hard-to-calculate-experts-weigh-in)

I will quote the next paragraphs from the article "Why are COVID-19 death rates so hard to calculate? Experts weigh in" they are crystal clear to me, and go in the same line of thoughts:

"Why 3.4% is likely an overestimate

Dr. Toni Ho, a consultant in infectious diseases at the Medical Research Council (MRC)–University of Glasgow Centre for Virus Research, U.K., echoes similar sentiments.

She goes on to suggest that the figure of 3.4% is likely an exaggeration, mainly due to the challenges of calculating mortality rates outlined above.

"The quoted mortality rate of 3.4% is taken from confirmed deaths over total reported cases. This is likely an overestimate, as a number of countries, such as the United States (112 confirmed, 10 deaths) and Iran (2,336 cases, 77 deaths), have had limited testing. Hence, few of the mild cases have been picked up, and [the total number of cases] we are observing is the tip of the iceberg."

In fact, the overestimation could be 10 times higher than the reality, notes Mark Woolhouse, a professor of Infectious Disease Epidemiology at the University of Edinburgh, U.K.

"If a significant number of mild cases have been missed or not reported, then this [3.4%] estimate is too high."

"Though there is disagreement about this, some studies have suggested that it is approximately 10 times too high. This would bring the death rate in line with some strains of influenza."

– Prof. Mark Woolhouse

COVID-19 Incubation Period

Recommended further reading:

https://www.worldometers.info/coronavirus/coronavirus-incubation-period/

The incubation period is the period from infection to the onset of symptoms.   As spreading might be possible, and apparently is, in asymptomatic patients, the duration of incubation period is a critical data necessary for the planning of containment measures. For example, to determine de suitable duration of quarantines. If you determine a shorter quarantine period than the actual incubation period, the enforced or self-imposed quarantine will possibly be useless. As some cases related to the Diamond Princess might prove.

According to the available data, COVID-19 incubation period is 2-14 days. But it could be as short as one day and as long as 27 days.

According to WHO and CDC, 2-14 days represents the current official estimated range for the novel coronavirus COVID-19. However, a case with an incubation period of 27 days has been reported by Hubei Province local government on Feb. 22. In addition, a case with an incubation period of 19 days was observed in a JAMA study of 5 cases published on Feb. 21. Another case of a 24 days incubation period had been for the first time observed in a Feb. 9 study. WHO said at the time that this could actually reflect a second exposure rather than a long incubation period, and that it wasn't going to change its recommendations. Anyways data confirm that Incubation Period can vary greatly among patients. Average incubation periods go from 3 days to 5.2 days according to different studies.

A Chinese study published in the New England Journal of Medicine on Jan. 30, has found the incubation period to be 5.2 days on average, but it varies greatly among patients. The Chinese team conducting the study said their findings support a 14-day medical observation period for people exposed to the pathogen.

Comparison with other viruses

For comparison, the incubation period for the common flu (seasonal influenza) is typically around 2 days. Incubation period for other coronaviruses: SARS 2-7 days; MERS 5 days typically (range 2-14 days).

COVID-19 and pets

A dog was tested weak positive for the virus in Hong Kong on February 26th. His owner was also a confirmed case. The result was considered at the moment as a possible environmental contamination. But two other posterior tests (on February 28th and March 2n also resulted weak positives again. The dog remains asymptomatic and quarantined. But the question remains open if pets, like children, although asymptomatic, might spread the disease.

Recommended further reading:

https://globalnews.ca/news/6608521/dog-quarantined-coronavirus

https://www.theguardian.com/world/2020/mar/05/hong-kong-warns-residents-not-to-kiss-pets-after-dog-contracts-coronavirus

COVID-19 Timeline

A Timeline is, in my opinion, one of the best ways to comprehend complex phenomena. Sadly, the items included in the list are chosen according to some, always arguable, criteria. I did my best to include the most relevant ones.

The data were collected on the web, in newspapers sites, and e-zines, and blogs.

For the first days of the outbreak, from December 1st on, I must credit Wikipedia outstanding and most interesting page. I extracted most relevant data, but it is really worth reading complete
https://en.wikipedia.org/wiki/Timeline_of_the_2019%E2%80%9320_coronav

And the World Health Organization releases daily Situation Reports you can read at the WHO site: https://www.who.int/emergencies/diseases/novel-coronavirus-2019/situation-reports

NOVEMBER 2019

As the first cases of COVID-19 were diagnosed by the first week of December, and considering an incubation period of a to 30 days, we can conclude that the patient zero should be located during the first two weeks of November.

DECEMBER 2019

2019/12/01-18 First registered cases lately recognized as COVID-19

On 31 December 2019, a consortium of Chinese medical experts was charged by the Chinese CDC with investigating the inception of what was commonly known as Wuhan coronavirus. On 24 January 2020, their report was published in The Lancet. They noted from their review of local medical records that the first person later to be diagnosed with the Wuhan coronavirus had first presented with symptoms on 8 December 2019. However, the consortium found an earlier case of a person who had first experienced symptoms on 1 December 2019, pointing to an even earlier origin. Apart from this early case, between 8 and 18 December 2019, seven cases later diagnosed with Wuhan coronavirus were documented, two of them were linked with the Huanan Seafood Wholesale Market of Wuhan, five were not.

2019/12/12 Chinese state broadcaster CCTV reported in a broadcast airing on 12 January 2020 that a "new viral outbreak was first detected in the city of Wuhan, China, on 12 December 2019."

2019/12/21 Chinese epidemiologists with the Chinese Center for Disease Control (CDC) published an article on 1 January 2020 stating that the first cluster of patients with "pneumonia of an unknown cause" had been identified on 21 December 2019.

2019/12/29 According to a CDC publication on 31 January 2020, the facts leading up to the identification of the 2019-nCoV were as follows, "On 29 December 2019, a hospital in Wuhan admitted four individuals with pneumonia and recognized that all four had worked in the Huanan Seafood Wholesale Market, which sells live poultry, aquatic products, and several kinds of wild animals to the public. The hospital reported this occurrence to the local center for disease control (CDC), which lead Wuhan CDC staff to initiate a field investigation with a retrospective search for pneumonia patients potentially linked to the market. The investigators found additional patients linked to the market, and on 30 December, health authorities from Hubei Province reported this cluster to China CDC. The following day, China CDC sent experts to Wuhan to support the investigation and control effort. Samples from these patients were obtained for laboratory analyses."

2019/12/30 On 30 December 2019, Dr. Li Wenliang, an ophthalmologist at Wuhan Central Hospital in Wuhan, China, posted a warning to alumni from his medical school class via a WeChat online forum that a cluster of seven patients treating within the ophthalmology department had been unsuccessfully treated for symptoms of viral pneumonia and diagnosed with SARS. Because these patients did not respond to traditional treatments, they were quarantined in an ER department of the Wuhan Central Hospital. In the WeChat forum, Li posted that this cluster of patients appeared to be infected by SARS. Dr. Li posted a snippet of an RNA analysis finding "SARS coronavirus" and extensive bacteria colonies in a patient's airways according to a chat transcript that he and other chat members later shared online. (Dr. Li contracted this coronavirus from a patient he treated, was hospitalized on 12 January 2020 and died on 6 February 2020. Due to public outcry directed to the CCP outlets retracted original reports, while international news agents corrected reports published on the 6th stating the death on 7th. The official date of death was later announced as 7 February 2020. Dr. Li is widely known for the statement he gave before his death exemplifying how the Chinese government botched the containment of the Wuhan coronavirus, stating "There should be more than one voice in a healthy society.")

The Chinese National Health Commission announced later that evening that eight doctors engaging in this WeChat forum had been arrested by Wuhan Police and charged with "illegal acts of fabricating, spreading rumors and disrupting social order..."

Wuhan medical authorities forbade doctors from making public announcements and ordered them to report cases internally.

News of an outbreak of "pneumonia of unknown origin" started circulating on social media on the evening of 30 December 2019. The social media reports stated that 27 patients in Wuhan - most of them stall holders at the Huanan Seafood Market - had been treated for the mystery illness.

On the evening of 30 December 2019, an "urgent notice on the treatment of pneumonia of unknown cause" was issued by the Wuhan Municipal Health Committee on its Weibo social media account. It was reported that since the beginning of December, there had been "a successive series of patients with unexplained pneumonia" - 27 suspected cases in total, seven of which were in critical condition and 18 were stable, two of which were on the verge of being discharged soon. The Wuhan Municipal Health Committee reported to the WHO that 27 people had been diagnosed with pneumonia of unknown cause. Most were stallholders from the Huanan Seafood Wholesale Market, seven of whom were in critical condition. The Wuhan Municipal Health Commission also made a public announcement regarding the situation.

Early investigations into the cause of the pneumonia ruled out seasonal flu, SARS, MERS and bird flu.

Hong Kong Secretary for Food and Health Sophia Chan Siu-Chee announced after an urgent night-time meeting with officials and experts, " [any suspected cases] including the presentation of fever and acute respiratory illness or pneumonia, and travel history to Wuhan within 14 days before onset of symptoms, we will put the patients in isolation."

2019/12/31 On 31 December 2019, an "urgent notice on the treatment of pneumonia of unknown cause" was issued to the Wuhan Municipal Health Center.

As a result of the official announcement of the Wuhan Municipal Health Commission, Hong Kong, Macau and Taiwan immediately tightened their inbound screening processes.

Qu Shiqian, a vendor at the Huanan Seafood Market, said government officials had disinfected the premises on 31 December 2019 and told stallholders to wear masks. Qu said he had only learnt of the pneumonia outbreak from media reports. "Previously I thought they had flu," he said. "It should be not serious. We are fish traders. How can we get infected?"

"Chinese state television reported that a team of experts from the National Health Commission had arrived in Wuhan on 31 December 2019 to lead the investigation, while the People's Daily said the exact cause remained unclear and it would be premature to speculate." Chinese state broadcaster CCTV reported that a team of senior health experts had been dispatched to the city of Wuhan and were reported to be "conducting relevant inspection and verification work."

Tao Lina, a public health expert and former official with Shanghai's Centre for disease control and prevention, said, "I think we are [now] quite capable of killing it in the beginning phase, given China's disease control system, emergency handling capacity and clinical medicine support."

2019/12/31 A pneumonia of unknown cause detected in Wuhan city was first reported to the WHO Country Office in China.

2020/01/01 Chinese health authorities close the Huanan Seafood Wholesale Market after it is discovered that wild animals sold there may be the source of the virus. According to the Chinese state-sponsored Xinhua News, the Huanan Seafood Market was closed on 1 January 2020 for "regulation." However, in the Consortium's report of 24 January 2020, it was stated that the Huanan Seafood Market had been closed on 1 January 2020 for "cleaning and disinfection."

JANUARY 2020

2020/01/01 Chinese Police accuses eight people, among them Dr. Li Wenliang, of spreading "false rumors" about a "new SARS-like virus". Later they would be referred to as "the eight brave (八勇士)" on some Chinese social media. Chinese police drop the case against them on January, 29th.

2020/01/03 Chinese scientists at the National Institute of Viral Disease Control and Prevention (IVDC) determined the genetic sequence of the novel β-genus coronaviruses (naming it '2019-nCoV') from specimens collected from patients in Wuhan, China, and three distinct strains were established.

Health authorities in Wuhan reported 44 cases, a big jump from the 27 reported on Tuesday. Eleven of the 44 were seriously ill, the Wuhan Municipal Health Commission said, although there had been no reported deaths to date. The health of the 121 close contacts of the cases was being monitored.

2020/01/03 Dr. Li Wenliang, the Wuhan ophthalmologist who had been arrested for spreading false "rumors" on WeChat, was summoned to the Wuhan Public Security Bureau where he was told to sign an official confession and admonition letter promising to cease spreading false "rumors" regarding the coronavirus. In the letter, he was accused of "making false comments" that had "severely disturbed the social order". The letter stated, "We solemnly warn you: If you keep being stubborn, with such impertinence, and continue this illegal activity, you will be brought to justice - is that understood?" Dr. Li signed the confession writing: "Yes, I understand." Li would later be supported e.g. in a blog run by China's Supreme People's Court on 28 January 2020. On 7 February 2020, Chinese state-sponsored news reported that Dr. Li had died from complications arising from his infection to the Wuhan coronavirus only to later delete the post and report Dr. Li as being in critical condition. He was subsequently confirmed the same day as having regrettably indeed deceased. Dr. Li is now being heralded as a whistleblower who exposed the Chinese government's early efforts to cover up the seriousness of the coronavirus pandemic which resulted in its rapid spread across China and the world.

2020/01/04 The head of the University of Hong Kong's Centre for Infection, Ho Pak-Leung, warned that the city should implement the strictest possible monitoring system for a mystery new viral pneumonia that infected dozens of people on the mainland, as it was highly possible that the illness was spreading from human to human. The microbiologist also warned that there could be a surge in cases during the upcoming Chinese New Year. Ho said he hoped the mainland would release more details as soon as possible about the patients infected with the disease, such as their medical history, to help experts analyze the illness and to allow for more effective preventive measures to be put in place.

The Singapore Ministry of Health said on Saturday, January 4, that it had been notified of the first suspected case of the "mystery Wuhan virus" in Singapore, involving a three-year-old girl from China who had pneumonia and a travel history to the Chinese city of Wuhan.On January 5, the

Singapore Ministry of Health released a press statement stating that the earlier suspected case was not linked to the pneumonia cluster in Wuhan and was also tested negative for the SARS and MERS-CoV.

Chinese officials were criticized for failing to disclose any information about the "mysterious virus" that machine translations of official reports suggested may be caused by a new coronavirus.

The WHO waited for China to release information about the "mysterious new pneumonia virus". The United Nations agency activated its incident-management system at the country, regional and global level and was standing ready to launch a broader response if it was needed. The WHO's regional office in Manila said in Twitter posts Saturday.: "#China has reported to WHO regarding a cluster of pneumonia cases in Wuhan, Hubei Province. The Government has also met with our country office, and updated @WHO on the situation. Government actions to control the incident have been instituted and investigations into the cause are ongoing."

The Wuhan Institute of Virology didn't respond to an emailed request for comment on the infectious source

2020/01/05 The number of suspected cases reached 59 with seven in a critical condition. All were quarantined and local medical officials commenced the monitoring of 163 of their contacts. At this time, there had been no reported cases of human-to-human transmission or presentations in healthcare workers.

2020/01/06 Chinese officials ruled out the possibility that this was a recurrence of the severe acute respiratory syndrome (SARS) virus - an illness that originated in China and killed more than 770 people worldwide in 2002-2003. The Wuhan health authorities announced they continued seeking the cause but had so far ruled out influenza, avian influenza, adenovirus, and coronaviruses SARS and MERS as the respiratory pathogen that had infected 59 people as of 5 January.

2020/01/06 The US Centers for Disease Control and Prevention (USCDC) issues a travel watch at Level 1 ("Practice usual precautions") with recommendations on washing hands and more specifically advising avoiding animals, animal markets, and contact with unwell people if travelling to Wuhan

2020/01/07 Since the outburst of social media discussion of the mysterious pneumonia outbreak in Wuhan, China, Chinese authorities censored the hashtag #WuhanSARS and were now investigating anyone who was allegedly spreading misleading information about the outbreak on social media.

2020/01/07 "The U.S. Centers for Disease Control and Prevention (CDC) issued a travel notice Monday for travelers to Wuhan, Hubei province, China due to the cluster of cases of pneumonia of an unknown etiology...

2020/01/08 Chinese scientist identify the new pathogen as a virus of the coronavirus family, like SARS and common cold viruses. They name it "2019-nCoV".

2020/01/09 Chinese scientists reported on Chinese state broadcaster CCTV that they had found a new "coronavirus in 15 of 57 patients with the illness in the central city of Wuhan, saying it has been preliminarily identified as the pathogen for the outbreak". The scientists announced that the current 'Wuhan Virus', a coronavirus, appears to not be as lethal as SARS. They reported that the new viral outbreak was first detected in the city of Wuhan on 12 December 2019. Additionally, a total of 59 people have been identified as contracting the illness, seven patients had been in a critical condition at some stage, and no healthcare workers were reported as having been infected.

2020/01/10 The gene sequencing data of the isolated 2019-nCoV, a virus from the same family as the SARS coronavirus, was posted on Virological.org by researchers from Fudan University, Shanghai. A further three sequences from the Chinese Center for Disease Control and Prevention, one from the Chinese Academy of Medical Sciences, and one from Jin Yintan Hospital in Wuhan were posted to the Global Initiative on Sharing All Influenza Data (GISAID) portal. The same day, Public Health England issued its guidance.

2020/01/10 Dr. Li Wenliang, Chinese ophthalmologist and coronavirus whistleblower, started having symptoms of a dry cough. On 12 January 2020, Dr. Wenliang started having a fever. He was admitted to the hospital on 14 January 2020. His parents also contracted the coronavirus (presumably from Dr. Wenliang) and were admitted to the hospital with him. Dr. Wenliang tested negative several times for the coronavirus until finally testing positive on 30 January 2020.

2020/01/11 China reports the first death from the novel disease. A sixty-one years old man, who had shopped at the Wuhan Market, died on January 9 after respiratory failure caused by severe pneumonia.

2020/01/17 Public Health Screening to Begin at 3 U.S. Airports for 2019 Novel Coronavirus ("2019-nCoV").

The CDC statement reads:

"The Centers for Disease Control and Prevention (CDC) and the Department of Homeland Security's Customs and Border Protection (CBP) will implement enhanced health screenings to detect ill travelers traveling to the United States on direct or connecting flights from Wuhan, China. This activity is in response to an outbreak in China caused by a novel (new) coronavirus (2019 nCoV), with exported cases to Thailand and Japan.

Starting January 17, 2020, travelers from Wuhan to the United States will undergo entry screening for symptoms associated with 2019-nCoV at three U.S. airports that receive most of the travelers from Wuhan, China: San Francisco (SFO), New York (JFK), and Los Angeles (LAX) airports."

2020/01/18 Wuhan City government held an annual banquet in the Baibuting community celebrating the Chinese New Year with forty thousand families in attendance despite the officials' knowledge of the spread of the Wuhan coronavirus. They shared meals, plates and ate together. On 21 January 2020 when Wuhan mayor Zhou Xianwang was asked on state television why this banquet was held even after the number of cases had risen to 312 he responded, "The reason why the Baibuting community continued to host the banquet this year was based on the previous judgment that the spread of the epidemic was limited between humans, so there was not enough warning."

2020/01/20 Scientists from the China CDC identified three different strains of the 2019-nCoV confirming that the original Wuhan coronavirus had mutated into two additional strains.

2020/01/20 Virus spreads outside China. Thailand and Japan report cases of infections in people who had visited the same Wuhan Market.

2020/01/20 First case reported in South Korea.

2020/01/20 The National Institutes of Health announces that it is working on a vaccine against the coronavirus. "The NIH is in the process of taking the first steps towards the development of a vaccine," says Dr. Anthony Fauci, director of the National Institutes of Allergy and Infectious Diseases.

2020/01/20 Officials confirm the virus can be passed directly between humans.

2020/01/20 Sales Meeting at the Grand Hyatt Hotel in Singapore. January 20-22. Five attendees of an as-yet-unnamed private international sales company meeting of 109 attendees, 94 from overseas, held from January 20–22 at the Grand Hyatt Hotel, Singapore were diagnosed with the Wuhan coronavirus upon returning home: one from Malaysia, two from South Korea and two from Singapore. One of the attendees was from Wuhan, China. It was reported that the company held a buffet for their delegates. These four diagnoses were not reported until February 5, 2020. The first laboratory-confirmed case in Singapore of an unrelated 67 years-old native of Wuhan was not reported until 23 January 2020. These cases linked to the meeting were the first evidence that the Wuhan coronavirus had spread through human-to-human contact outside China, which the WHO has said is deeply concerning and could signal evidence of a much larger outbreak. As of February 5, 2020, the sister of a Malaysian who attended the meeting had been infected and four more local staff in Singapore were confirmed as having virus symptoms.

2020/01/21 A total of 291 cases have now been reported across major cities in China, including Beijing and Shanghai. However, most patients are in Wuhan, the central city of 11 million at the heart of the outbreak.

2020/01/21 A report by the MRC Centre for Global Infectious Disease Analysis at Imperial College London suggested there could be more than 1,700 infections. However, Gabriel Leung, the dean of medicine at the University of Hong Kong, put the figure closer to 1,300.

2020/01/21 After 300 confirmed diagnoses and 6 deaths, Chinese state media warned lower-level officials not to cover up the spread of a new coronavirus. Officials declared that anyone who concealed new cases would "be nailed on the pillar of shame for eternity", the political body responsible for law and order said. Local Chinese officials initially withheld information about the epidemic from the public. It later vastly under-reported the number of people that had been infected, downplayed the risks and failed to provide timely information that experts say could have saved lives. In its commentary published online on Tuesday January 20, 2020, the Communist Party's Central Political and Legal Commission talked of China having learned a "painful lesson" from the SARS epidemic and called for the public to be kept informed. Deception, it warned, could "turn a controllable natural disaster into a man-made disaster".

2020/01/21 The Wuhan Municipal Health Commission reported at least 15 medical workers in Wuhan have also been infected with the virus, with one in a critical condition.

2020/01/21 The World Health Organization releases WHO Situation Report 1: (Please note that the WHO Situation Reports as official reportage stand on their own.)

Confirmed cases were reported in several new locations in China. Zhejiang province and Tianjin reported five and two laboratory-confirmed cases, respectively. Guangdong reported three additional laboratory-confirmed cases. Shanghai and Henan province reported an additional four and one laboratory-confirmed cases, respectively. One laboratory-confirmed case was reported in Sichuan province, and Chongqing reported five laboratory-confirmed cases. Shandong, Hunan, and Yunnan all reported one laboratory-confirmed case each. Jiangxi reported two laboratory-confirmed cases. The total number of laboratory-confirmed cases in China increased to 312 and the death toll increased to six.

2020/01/21 New cases were also reported outside of mainland China. Taiwan reported its first laboratory-confirmed case, and the United States reported its first laboratory-confirmed case in the state of Washington, the first in North America. https://www.infectioncontroltoday.com/hai-types/coronavirus-case-confirmed-washington-state

2020/01/21 China's Wuhan Institute filed to patent the use of Gilead's Remdesivir for the treatment of novel coronavirus.

2020/01/22 Millions under lockdown. Chinese Government decrees quarantine on Hunan city, home of eleven million people, to commence 23 January 2020 at 10:00 am. No traffic will be allowed in or out of the city. Officials eventually extend quarantine to thirteen other cities in Hubei and Hunan states affecting more than thirty-six million people. However, statistics compiled by the Chinese Railway Administration showed that on the same day approximately 100,000 people had already departed from Wuhan Train Station by the deadline. Furthermore, many Wuhan residents bypassed the checkpoints by taking antipyretics, having seen tips shared on Sina Weibo.

2020/01/22 North Korea closed its borders and banned foreign tourists over the virus.

2020/01/23 WHO states it is too early to declare a Global Public Health Emergency. However, new cases of infection are confirmed outside China, in several countries, including South Korea, United States, Nepal, Thailand, Hong Kong, Singapore, Malaysia and Taiwan.

2020/01/23 Wuhan suspended all public transportation from 10 a.m. onwards, including all bus, metro and ferry lines. Additionally, all outbound trains and flights were halted.

2020/01/24 Second imported case reported by the United States CDC. The patient returned to the U.S. from Wuhan on January 13, 2020, and called a health care provider after experiencing symptoms a few days later. The case eleven days after the patient arrived to the United States. https://www.cdc.gov/media/releases/2020/p0124-second-travel-coronavirus.html

2020/01/24 CoVid-19 reaches Europe and Australia. The first three cases in Europe are reported by France.

2020/01/24 The first confirmed incidence of human-to-human transmission outside of China was documented by the WHO in Vietnam.

2020/01/24 A study by Chinese researchers indicates that people can be symptom-free for several days while the coronavirus is incubating, increasing the risk of contagious infection without forewarning signs.

2020/01/24 By the end of the day, the entire Hubei province had gone under a city-by-city quarantine, apart from Xiangyang and Shennongjia Forestry District.

2020/01/24 All 70,000 Chinese cinemas were closed until further notice. Multiple tourist sites across China were closed until further notice, including Mount Wutai, Pingyao, Yanmen Pass, Xuanwu Lake, Qixia Mountain, Nanking Massacre Museum, Sun Yat-sen Memorial Hall, Canton Tower, Gulangyu, Yu Garden, Shanghai Disneyland, West Lake, and Forbidden City.

2020/01/24 The Beijing and Shanghai governments have "urged residents returning from coronavirus outbreak areas to stay at home for 14 days to prevent its spread."

2020/01/24 Citing the coronavirus outbreak, Starbucks and McDonald's suspended some operations in China.

2020/01/25 Chinese Communist Party general secretary Xi Jinping called the "accelerating spread" of the coronavirus a "grave situation" in a Party Politburo meeting, and that it was "mutating" as Beijing escalates measures to contain the illness.

2020/01/25 Chinese Lunar New Year holiday is extended by three days. Officials cancel many major public events. By late January, seventeen Chinese cities, home of more than fifty million people, are under lockdown. Beijing announced it will halt all inter-provincial bus and train services starting 26 January.

2020/01/25 Borders Closed. Mongolia, Hong Kong and Russia close their borders with China.

2020/01/25 Australia confirmed its first four cases, one in Victoria and three in New South Wales. Malaysia reported its first three cases in Johor Bahru, and a fourth case later. Japan confirmed its third case. Canada confirmed its first case in Toronto. Thailand added two new cases for a total of seven. Singapore confirmed fourth case.

2020/01/25 Hong Kong declared a state of emergency. and announced it would close schools until 17 February. Hong Kong Disneyland and Ocean Park are closed until further notice.

2020/01/26 China started requiring nationwide use of monitoring stations for screening, identification and immediate isolation of coronavirus-infected travelers, including at airports, railway stations, bus stations and ports. Schools in Beijing would stay closed until further notice to prevent further spread of the coronavirus. Separately, the Beijing Government stated it will not lock-down the city.

2020/01/26 A tentative clinical profile for the new coronavirus (2019-nCoV) was published by an assistant professor of population health science at the Icahn School of Medicine at Mount Sinai in New York. The lethality of the virus is unknown; however, the death toll has now climbed to above three digits.

2020/01/27 The USCDC expands travel advisory from Wuhan to the whole of Hubei Province. Later that day, the US State Department raised the travel advisory for China to Level 3 ("Reconsider Travel: Avoid travel due to serious risks to safety and security.") due to the coronavirus. The same day, the USCDC again updates its travel health notice to Warning - Level 3, Avoid All Nonessential Travel to China.

2020/01/27 Dr. Gabriel Leung, Dean of the University of Hong Kong medical school and one of the foremost world experts on SARS and viruses, gave a three-hour presentation published on YouTube wherein he made now casts and forecasts of the coronavirus. Using traditional scientific modeling techniques that predict the spread of viruses, Dr. Leung projected the true number of coronavirus infections was likely 10 time more than the official reported numbers. Dr. Leung estimated that there were between 44,000-100,000 infections in China as of 24 January 2020. He stated that draconian measures were needed to slow the progress of the virus but that these measures would have no effect in stopping the coronavirus pandemic. He projected that the number of infections would continue exponentially peeking out in late April or May 2020. Dr. Leung predicted that at the peak of the pandemic, there could be up to 100,000 new infections per day. Dr. Leung subsequently published an article in The Lancet now casting and forecasting the likely progression of the Wuhan coronavirus taking into consideration numerous variables.

2020/01/27 Xian Yang city announced the suspension of ferry services at 00:00 on 28 January, putting the entirety of Hubei province under a city-by-city quarantine, save for Shennongjia Forestry District. The move came after the closure of its railway stations at 00:00 on 27 January, and shutting down of its airport and inter-city bus services earlier.

2020/01/27 Wuhan suspends visa and passports services for Chinese citizens until 30 January.

2020/01/27 The Shanghai government said companies in the city are not allowed to resume operations before 9 February. Chinese tech company Tencent asks staff to work from home until 7 February due to coronavirus.

2020/01/27 Zhou Xianwang, the mayor of Wuhan, acknowledges criticism over his handling of the crisis, admitting that information was not released quickly enough. He said he would resign if it helped with public opinion but pointed out the local government was obliged to seek permission before fully disclosing information about the virus. Wuhan mayor said on a Chinese state television talk show that rules imposed by Beijing limited what he could disclose about the threat posed by the Wuhan coronavirus as it unfolded, suggesting "the central government was partially responsible for a lack of transparency that has marred the response to the fast-expanding health crisis."

2020/01/27 In Germany, the first specific, global case of coronavirus being transmitted by a person with no symptoms has been reported. The originally-infected individual is from Shanghai.

2020/01/27 Japan, Taiwan and Germany report first cases of domestic transmission. In China death toll reaches 132, and there are above six thousand reported infected worldwide.

2020/01/28 China's Supreme People's Court ruled that whistleblower, Li Wenliang, had not committed the crime of spreading "rumors" when on 30 December 2019 he posted to a WeChat forum for medical school alumni that seven patients under his care appeared to have contracted SARS. In their ruling, the Supreme People's Court stated, "If society had at the time believed those 'rumors', and wore masks, used disinfectant and avoided going to the wildlife market as if there were a SARS outbreak, perhaps it would've meant we could better control the coronavirus today," the court said. "Rumors end when there is openness."

2020/01/28 International evacuation begins. Japan and the United States are the first countries to evacuate some of their citizens from Wuhan. Australia and New Zealand announce evacuation plans too.

2020/01/28 A UK-Chinese medical research paper reports a statistical model finding that "estimates suggest the actual number of infected cases could be much higher than the reported, with estimated 26,701 cases (as of 28th January 2020)."

2020/01/28 Scientists from The Peter Doherty Institute for Infection and Immunity (Doherty Institute) in Melbourne reported that they had successfully grown 2019-nCoV from a patient sample.

2020/01/29 The White House announces the formation of a new task force that will help monitor and contain the spread of the virus, and ensure Americans have accurate and up-to-date health and travel information, it said.

2020/01/29 Companies in Hubei are required not to resume services before 13 February, and schools in Hubei are to postpone reopening.

2020/01/29 Chinese police drop their case against eight people, accused on 1 January of spreading "false rumors" about a "new SARS-like virus"; they have been referred to as "the eight brave (八勇士)" on some Chinese social media.

2020/01/29 Twitter Public Policy declares: We want to help you access credible information, especially when it comes to public health. We've adjusted our search prompt in key countries across the globe to feature authoritative health sources when you search for terms related to novel #coronavirus.

2020/01/29 United Arab Emirates Confirmed First Cases of the New Coronavirus in the Middle East. Coronavirus cases in UAE to be treated free of cost, insurance not necessary. UAE ministry issues new guidelines for schools on coronavirus. Any student, staff or associated family member who has flown in from China in the past 14 days, is to be exempted from school. The UAE's civil aviation authority has announced that all flights to and from the People's Republic of China (with the exception of Beijing) will be suspended as of February 5, 2020 until further notice.

2020/01/29 British Airways and Lufthansa cancel all flights to and from mainland China.

2020/01/30 The United States reports first case of domestic transmission.

The Centers for Disease Control and Prevention (CDC) has confirmed its first case of person-to-person transmission.

2020/01/30 The US State Department issued an updated travel advisory as "Level 4: Do Not Travel to China." Its website stated that "Those currently in China should consider departing" and warning that "Travelers should be prepared for travel restrictions to be put into effect with little or no advance notice". Additionally, it authorized American diplomatic staff and their families to evacuate China.

2020/01/30 Inter-provincial charter cars in mainland China and inter-provincial passenger routes to Hubei have all been suspended. Passenger transport on roads in ten provinces and municipalities including Hubei and Beijing has been suspended, inter-provincial passenger trains have been suspended in 16 provinces, urban bus routes have been suspended or partially suspended in multiple cities in 28 provinces, and urban rail transportation has been suspended in 5 cities including Wuhan.

2020/01/30 The Huanggang Communist Party committee announced the dismissal of its health chief, Tang Zhihong.

2020/01/30 The outbreak was declared a Public Health Emergency of

International Concern by the WHO. However, WHO Secretary-General, Dr. Tedros Adhanom Ghebreysus does not recommend trade and travel restrictions, saying these would be "an unnecessary disruption".

2020/01/30 Facebook publicly commits to limit the spread of misinformation and harmful content about the virus and to connect people to helpful information.

2020/01/30 Air France and KLM cancel all flights to mainland China until February 9.

2020/01/30 Two K-pop concerts in Singapore by Taeyeon and NCT Group respectively were postponed after the virus situation worsened.

2020/01/31 Russia, Spain, Sweden and the United Kingdom confirmed their first cases of the virus.

2020/01/31 China National Railway Group announced that starting 1 February, rail ticket purchases must provide the traveler's mobile phone number (email address for foreigners).

2020/01/31 The United States government declares a Public Health Emergency due to the coronavirus, and is closing its borders to all foreign nationals "who pose a threat of transmitting the virus from entering the country and would quarantine U.S. citizens returning from Hubei province in China, the epicenter of the outbreak, for up to 14 days," starting Sunday, February 2 at 5 p.m. The 195 Americans on the Air Force base in California whom were recently evacuated from Wuhan recently will also be quarantined.

2020/01/31 Chinese health experts warn the public that coronavirus patients can become re-infected. China starts repatriating citizens to Wuhan.

FEBRUARY 2020

2020/02/01 New cases were confirmed in Australia, Canada, Germany, Japan, Singapore, the US, the UAE and Vietnam.

2020/02/01 The Ministry of Ecology and Environment issued a notice late in the evening to deploy medical wastewater and urban sewage supervision, regulate emergency medical wastewater treatment, sterilization and disinfection requirements, in order to prevent the spread of new coronavirus through feces and sewage, after the feces of a patient was tested positive for the virus in Shenzhen.

2020/02/01 The Department of Civil Affairs of Hubei Province suspends all marriage registrations starting on 3 February 2020.

2020/02/01 Hubei implements a much stricter control, allowing only one person from each household every two days to be on the street for purchases, unless for medically-related reasons, required for epidemic control, or as shop workers.

2020/02/01 Alibaba Group announced free taxi service for health professionals in Wuhan.

2020/02/01 Hunan government required companies in the province not to resume business before 24:00 on 9 February; the new semester is not to start earlier than 17 February for primary and secondary schools and kindergartens, and 24 February for post-secondary institutions. Tianjin government issued a notice to postpone business resumption and the start of the new semester.

2020/02/01 China Federation of Radio and Television Associations issued a notice to pause the filming of all films and TV dramas in mainland China during the epidemic.

2020/02/01 Apple Inc. temporarily closed all Apple Stores in mainland China until 24:00 on 9 February.

2020/02/01 China's National Health Commission (NHC) announced new regulations Saturday requiring that all who lose their lives to the coronavirus must be cremated at the nearest facility. "No farewell ceremonies or other funeral activities involving the corpse shall be held," according to the new ruling.

2020/02/02 First death outside China reported in Philippines. A Chinese man from Wuhan who died of pneumonia.

2020/02/02 Prevention and Control HQ issued a set of traditional Chinese medicine (TCM) prescriptions "to help treat the infection". This move follows the 22 January recommendation from the National Health Commission to use TCM to treat the disease. The same official file that contains the prescription also demands that all patients in Wuhan be treated by TCM.

2020/02/02 With immediate effect, Wuhan's government announced the quarantining of "all suspected patients and those known to have been in close contact with a confirmed case." It stated "Patients shall cooperate. Whoever refuses to cooperate will be subject to enforcement by the police.

2020/02/02 China global automakers have already extended factory closures in line with government guidelines. Those manufacturers include Hyundai, Tesla, Ford, PSA Peugeot Citroen, Nissan and Honda Motors.

2020/02/03 The Chinese New Year holiday period ended after having been extended for a week. Mainland stock exchanges reopened, Shanghai Stock Exchange falling by 7.72% and Shenzhen Stock Exchange by 8.45%, with a total of 3,177 shares triggering the limit down of 10%. The RMB to USD exchange rate fell through 7.00, opening at 6.9249 and closing at 7.0257.

2020/02/03 Chinese government opens a new one thousand and six hundred beds Hospital in Wuhan city. The Huo Shen Shan (Fire God Mountain) Hospital was built in just ten days.

2020/02/03 The Diamond Princess is quarantined in Yokohama, Japan. The Japanese Health Ministry announces that ten people aboard the Diamond Princess cruise ship moored in Yokohama Bay are confirmed to have the coronavirus. The ship, which is carrying more than 3,700 people, is placed under quarantine scheduled to end on February 19.

2020/02/04 The first case was confirmed in Belgium in a person who was repatriated from Wuhan.

2020/02/05 The first shelter hospital is put into use. Designated hospitals in Wuhan will now accept only serious cases (confirmed or suspected); other existing and future patients would be redirected to shelter hospitals or community quarantine points

2020/02/05 Eighty Russian citizens evacuated by plane and set under quarantine, thus far no infections were identified. Russia sets up a quarantine area in Siberia's Tyumen region for Russians being evacuated from the epicenter of the coronavirus outbreak. All evacuated citizens will be held in quarantine for 14 days.

2020/02/06 Shipping of CDC 2019 Novel Coronavirus Diagnostic Test Kits Begins

Distribution of CDC Diagnostic Test Kits Will Expand Laboratory

Capacity to Detect 2019-nCoV

A CDC-developed laboratory test kit to detect 2019 novel coronavirus (2019-nCoV) began shipping yesterday to select qualified U.S. and international laboratories. Distribution of the tests will help improve the global capacity to detect and respond to the 2019 novel coronavirus.

The test kit, called the Centers for Disease Control and Prevention (CDC) 2019-Novel Coronavirus (2019-nCov) Real-Time Reverse Transcriptase (RT)-PCR Diagnostic Panel (CDC 2019-nCoV Real Time RT-PCR), is designed for use with an existing RT-PCR testing instrument that is commonly used to test for seasonal influenza.

The CDC 2019 novel coronavirus test is intended for use with upper and lower respiratory specimens collected from people who meet CDC criteria for 2019-nCoV testing. The test uses a technology that can provide results in four hours from initial sample processing to result.

Initially, about 200 test kits will be distributed to U.S. domestic laboratories and a similar amount will be distributed to select international laboratories. Each test kit can test approximately 700 to 800 patient specimens.

2020/02/07 Wuhan Central Hospital announces on Weibo (Chinese social network, a Twitter-like website) that Li Wenliang, the 34 years old Chinese doctor who was the first to warn colleagues about the novel disease, died at 2.58 a.m. despite attempts to resuscitate him.

The phrase "We want freedom of speech" begins to trend on Weibo, a Twitter-like website, before it is censored by the platform. Weibo users soon after create another hashtag: "I want freedom of speech", which quickly draws nearly 2 million views.

Vigils were held in Hong Kong and Wuhan to mourn Li Wenliang, an ophthalmologist at Wuhan Central Hospital who sounded the alarm on the coronavirus, for which Chinese authorities attempted to silence him. Wenliang died after contracting the virus.

The big picture, according New York Times' Li Yuan: "For many people in China, the doctor's death shook loose pent-up anger and frustration at how the government mishandled the situation by not sharing information earlier and by silencing whistle-blowers."

The Chinese government delayed a concerted public health offensive around the coronavirus by silencing doctors for raising red flags in the first seven weeks after first cases appeared in Wuhan city, in December.

2020/02/07 Hangzhou imposed a temporary ban on retail pharmacies selling fever and cough medicines, asking citizens with the symptoms to see a doctor instead.

2020/02/09 Coronavirus global death toll surpasses SARS. The novel coronavirus, 2019-nCoV, has now killed more people than the 2003 SARS outbreak.

2020/02/09 Chinese government opens a second prefabricated hospital with 1,600 beds in Wuhan to treat patients infected with coronavirus.

2020/02/10 President Xi Jinping appeared in public for the first time since the epidemic began, wearing a protective mask and his temperature was checked while visiting a hospital in Beijing and urging confidence in the battle against the virus.

2020/02/10 Business has now resumed in all 30 mainland province-level divisions, apart from Hubei.

2020/02/10 Food prices in China have risen on month of January. According to the consumer price index (CPI) the price of pork rose 8.5%, while the CPI came in at 5.4%. The reason may be due to food hoarding, besides the disruptions of supply chains due to transportation, lockdown measures and holiday demand. The CPI is the highest since October 2011.

2020/02/10 Tibetan New Year public activities due to occur on 24 February were suspended due to the Coronavirus disease 2019 epidemic. Praying activities inside monasteries in Lhasa will be held but will be shortened, without the participation of the public and in a smaller scale.

2020/02/11 WHO gives name to new coronavirus disease

The World Health Organization has officially named the disease caused by the new coronavirus as 'Covid-19'.

2020/02/11 Shenzhen University announced the successful development of a new coronavirus antibody detection kit capable of obtaining a result in 22 minutes and reducing the risk of infection of medical staff.

2020/02/12 Mobile World Congress cancelled

The largest global mobile event, Mobile World Congress, has been cancelled over coronavirus fears. The decision is said to be based on 'the global concern regarding the coronavirus outbreak, travel concern and other circumstances'. This comes after various exhibitors, including Facebook, Amazon, Sony, Nokia and LG said that they would be pulling out of the event. It was to take place in Barcelona, in February. The 2019 edition of the Mobile World Congress was attended by over a hundred thousand visitors.

2020/02/12 Airbnb suspended booking in Beijing until 30 April.

2020/02/13 Wuhan city enacts a new rule prohibiting people from leaving their neighborhoods for non-medical reasons.

2020/02/13 Japan reports first Covid-19 death. Japan health minister Katsunobu Kato confirmed the first Covid-19 death in the country – a woman in her 80s whose infection was reported to have been confirmed after death.

The total number of cases in Japan reached 248, including 218 from the quarantined cruise ship and 30 in the country.

2020/02/13 North Korea imposed a month-long quarantine on all foreign visitors and others suspected to have COVID-19.

2020/02/14 The central districts of Yunmeng County in Xiaogan, Hubei entered wartime control. Huanggang, Hubei escalated control starting 00:00, prohibiting non-essential persons or vehicles from entering and exiting communities and initiating the organized distribution of basic necessities.

2020/02/14 A new test kit was developed by a team led by Zhong Nanshan, able to yield a result in fifteen minutes with a very high sensitivity and expected to raise the positive detection rate.

2020/02/14 Beijing required all persons returning to the city to self-quarantine for 14 days.

2020/02/14 Shenzhen Metro would start using real-name system starting February 16th for epidemic tracing, with passengers able to self-register the carriages they ride in by scanning the QR code in the train.

2020/02/14 France reported Europe's first death from the virus.

2020/02/14 Egypt announces its first case of Wuhan coronavirus on Friday, according to a joint statement by Egypt's Ministry of Health and the WHO. The confirmed case marks the first in Africa since the virus was detected.

2020/02/14 Passengers on Westerdam cruise ship disembark. Westerdam cruise ship, which docked in Cambodia after being turned away by five countries over the fear of the coronavirus, has received permission to disembark its guests after 20 samples taken onboard tested negative.

2020/02/14 Honghu city, in Hubei, entered wartime control at 00:00, the decision announced during the day before evening.

Jingmen city, also in Hubei, escalated control, prohibiting outside vehicles and persons from entering its central districts except for medical and living supplies, and shutting down all business except approved pharmacies, supermarkets, and hotels.

2020/02/16 Taiwan recorded its first death of a taxi driver in his 60s due to the coronavirus.

2020/02/16 Hubei implements "hard quarantine" in rural villages; no outsiders are to be allowed in, and each household is allowed one person every three days to go out for provisions and urgent agricultural material, on designated routes and for limited time. All nonessential public spaces in Hubei are to be closed and all gatherings forbidden. Following its decision on the previous day, the city of Wuxue in Huang Gang now bans residents and vehicles from the streets. Those found to be not compliant are to be sent to a stadium for "centralized compulsory study" and their cars confiscated.

2020/02/16 In response to allegations that patient zero was its research student, Wuhan Institute of Virology released a statement saying no members of the Institute was infected and that the student had been working in other provinces for years.

2020/02/17 More than 450 confirmed cases out of 3700 passengers and crew in the Diamond Princess.

2020/02/17 Following its announcement the previous night, Xiaogan city bans all urban residents from leaving home, and all rural residents from wandering, visiting neighbors, and gathering, and all vehicles from roads. Exceptions are made for medical reasons, medical staff, providers of medical and living provision, pregnancies, deaths, essential vehicles, and others granted permissions. Violators would be subject to up to 10 days of detention and put on the dishonest list

2020/02/18 China's daily infection figures drop below 2,000 for the first time since January, with the country's health commission reporting 72,436 infections on the mainland and 1,868 deaths.

2020/02/18 Russia bans entry for Chinese citizens from February 20.

2020/02/19 Wuhan bans all particular vehicles from roads.

2020/02/19 Iranian Government reports two deaths in the city of Qom. The outbreak appears to have started there, in Qom, located about two hours from Tehran. The city of Qom is also home to the Fatima Masoumeh shrine, which draws pilgrims from all over the world.

2020/02/19 Passengers on Diamond Princess disembark. Passengers who have tested negative started disembarking from the cruise ship after a 14-day quarantine period, despite mounting evidence from infectious disease experts they could unknowingly be carrying the virus back into their communities.

2020/02/20 Hubei requires businesses in the province not to resume before 10 March, except for essential industries. Wenzhou removed all checkpoints except in Yueqing and reopened highways.

2020/02/20 Wuhan requires residents to measure their temperature twice daily and report any measurements exceeding 37.3 °C (99.1 °F).

2020/02/21 Three cases confirmed in Italy. A dozen towns, most of them just south of Milan in lockdown.

2020/02/21 Israel reported its first confirmed case of the coronavirus after a woman who returned from a cruise ship tested positive.

2020/02/21 Ukraine protesters attack China evacuee buses

Protesters in a Ukrainian town have attacked buses carrying evacuees from China. The evacuees were being transported to a hospital in Novi Sanzhary. All evacuees tested negative during official screening. The protest comes after a fake email, which was claimed to be from the Ministry of Health, said some evacuees had contracted the virus. Ukraine's security service (SSU) said that the false email is being investigated. According to media reports, nine police and one civilian were hospitalized, while more than ten protesters were detained.

2020/02/21 More than 500 cases confirmed in five prisons in Hubei, Shandong, and Zhejiang. Following the news of the outbreak, the responsible officials in Shandong and Hubei were dismissed. Henan and Shandong removed all road quarantine measures. Gansu adjusts its emergency response level for COVID-19 from level 1 to level 3.

Following some public confusion with the data released, Hubei prohibited the subtraction of clinically diagnosed cases. A corrected province-wide statistical report was available late in the evening.

Wuhan finished the testing of all existing suspected patients, patients with fever, and people with close contact.

2020/02/22 Wuhan requires a 14-day quarantine for patients discharged from COVID-19.

2020/02/22 2020 growth for China would be 5.6 percent. This is 0.4 percentage points lower than the January WEO Update. Global growth would be about 0.1 percentage points lower.

Remarks by IMF Managing Director Kristalina Georgieva to G20 on Economic Impact of COVID-19

February 22, 2020

Today in Riyadh, Ms. Kristalina Georgieva, Managing Director of the International Monetary Fund (IMF), made the following statement at the G20 Finance Ministers and Central Bank Governors Meeting:

"In January, we projected global growth to strengthen from 2.9 percent last year to 3.3 percent this year. Since then, COVID-19—a global health emergency—has disrupted activity in China. And let me say here that my deepest sympathies go to the people in China and other affected countries.

"The Chinese authorities are working to mitigate the negative impact on the economy, with crisis measures, liquidity provision, fiscal measures, and financial support. I have had an excellent discussion with Governor Yi Gang and other senior officials and assured them of our support for these policy measures.

"While the impact of the epidemic continues to unfold, the WHO's assessment is that with strong and coordinated measures, the spread of the virus in China and globally can yet be contained and the human tragedy arrested. We are still learning about how this complex virus spreads and the uncertainties are too great to permit reliable forecasting. Many scenarios can play out, depending on how quickly the virus is contained and how fast the Chinese and other affected economies return to normal.

"In our current baseline scenario, announced policies are implemented and China's economy would return to normal in the second quarter. As a result, the impact on the world economy would be relatively minor and short-lived.

"In this scenario, 2020 growth for China would be 5.6 percent. This is 0.4 percentage points lower than the January WEO Update. Global growth would be about 0.1 percentage points lower.

"But we are also looking at more dire scenarios   where the spread of the virus continues for longer and more globally, and the growth consequences   are   more protracted.

"Global cooperation is essential to the containment of the COVID-19 and its economic impact, particularly if the outbreak turns out to be more persistent and widespread. To be adequately prepared, now is the time to recognize the potential risk for fragile states and countries with weak health care systems.

"The IMF stands ready to   help,   including through our Catastrophe Containment and Relief Trust that can provide grants for debt relief to our poorest and most vulnerable members." https://www.imf.org/en/News/Articles/2020/02/22/pr2061-remarks-by-kristalina-georgieva-to-g20-on-economic-impact-of-covid-19

2020/02/23 At the G20 Finance Ministers and Central Bank Governors Meeting in Riyadh, finance ministers and central bank governors of the world's largest countries pledged to "enhance global risk monitoring" and warned the coronavirus posed a serious threat to global growth.

2020/02/24 Fears for the spread of the coronavirus in northern Italy have caused all public events, included the Venice carnival, to be canceled, and schools and museums in Lombardy, Veneto and Piedmont are closed until March, 1st.

2020/02/24 Iran official states 50 deaths in the country on February 13th; government denies claims. ILNA news agency quoted a Qom city official named Ahmad Amiriabadi Farahani as saying that the death toll in the country stood at 50 on February 13th (eleven days ago). However, the officials have stated on 24 February that death toll increased only up to twelve. Iran's Deputy Health Minister Iraj Harirchi has rejected the claims of cover-up. He stated that it was 'not the time for political confrontations'. Farahani denied to retract his statement.

2020/02/24 Coronavirus stress tests American drug industry's dependence on China.

"It's unclear whether the rapid spread of the novel coronavirus will actually result in prescription drug shortages, but it has undoubtedly highlighted the potential vulnerabilities of having the supply chain for American drugs so dependent on China.

Driving the news: About 150 prescription drugs — including antibiotics, generics and some branded drugs without alternatives — are at risk of shortage if the coronavirus outbreak in China worsens, per two sources familiar with a list of at-risk drugs compiled by the Food and Drug Administration.

China is a huge supplier of the ingredients used to make drugs that are sold in the U.S.

The FDA declined to comment on the list, but said in a statement that it's "keenly aware that the outbreak could impact the medical product supply chain" and has devoted additional resources toward identifying vulnerabilities to U.S. medical products.

What they're saying: In response to Axios' reporting, Sen. Josh Hawley will today send a letter to the FDA calling the degree of U.S. reliance on China for drugs "inexcusable."

"It is becoming clear to me that both oversight hearings and additional legislation are necessary to determine the extent of our reliance on Chinese production and protect our medical product supply chain," Hawley writes.

Flashback: Lawmakers have voiced concern before. Democratic Reps. Anna Eshoo and Adam Schiff — who chair the Energy and Commerce health subcommittee and the Intelligence Committee, respectively — wrote an op-ed in the Washington Post last year.

"Depending on any single supplier for such lifesaving goods would be troubling, but when that supplier is China at a time of rising tensions and conflict, it's a national security issue that demands the attention of the administration and Congress," they wrote." Read Caitlin Owens' full article in Axios.com https://www.axios.com/coronavirus-china-prescription-drugs-united-states-9342fa92-e8bd-4b67-8a7e-f8a4402988cb.html

2020/02/25 The NIH announces that a clinical trial to evaluate the safety and effectiveness of the antiviral drug Remdesivir in adults diagnosed with coronavirus has started at the University of Nebraska Medical Center in Omaha. The first participant is an American who was evacuated from the Diamond Princess cruise ship docked in Japan.

2020/02/25 First suspected case of community spread in the United States. Algeria reports first case; second African country with confirmed cases

2020/02/25 Algeria reported its first positive case – an Italian adult who arrived in the African country on 17 February. This represents the second case in Africa.

2020/02/25 Jamaica and the Cayman Islands denied entry to Meraviglia cruise ship as it carried a sick crew member who travelled to countries with confirmed coronavirus cases.

2020/02/25 Switzerland confirmed its first Covid-19 case in canton of Ticino. Swiss health ministry noted the man was in Italy approximately ten days ago when he attended an event near Milan.

2020/02/25 Brazil reports its first case of the coronavirus.

2020/02/25 Iran Deputy Health Minister tests positive; one more death reported. Iranian Deputy Health Minister Iraj Harirchi tested positive for the coronavirus, confirmed health ministry spokesman. Iran's Deputy Health Minister Iraj Harirchi had rejected the claims of cover-up just a day ago, on February 24th.

2020/02/25 Coronavirus disrupts sporting events around the world.

Four Serie A soccer matches in Northern Italy were canceled, and the government wants future games in areas affected by the outbreak to be played behind closed doors without fans.

Athletics: The World Athletics Indoor Championships, set to take place in mid-March in Nanjing, China, has been postponed until next year.

Formula One: The Chinese Grand Prix, originally scheduled for April 19 in Shanghai, has been postponed.

Table tennis: The world championship to be held in late March in South Korea has been pushed back provisionally to late June.

2020 Japan Olympic Games: Japanese officials insist the 2020 Tokyo Olympics will go on as planned, but the coronavirus has already begun to affect preparations. Movement of athletes has been limited, qualifying events have been disrupted, and plans to train tens of thousands of volunteers have been postponed. There are also emerging questions about how many people will be willing to travel to watch the Olympics. Coronavirus fears have led to a huge drop in tourism to Asia. Longtime International Olympic Committee member Dick Pound estimates that the IOC has until late May to decide if the Olympics can go forward as scheduled. In case IOC decides not to go forward as scheduled, the Games would be cancelled, not simply postponed. Despite previous disease outbreaks (Zika in 2014) and frequent geopolitical tensions, the Olympics have only been canceled three times, all due to world wars (1916, 1940, 1944).

"It's premature to call for the cancellation or postponement of Tokyo 2020. But with the torch relay about to begin and just 150 days remaining to the Opening Ceremonies, it's certainly not too early to ask how the organizers and the IOC realistically propose to keep the Summer Games healthy and secure."

"How can they prevent an outbreak with athletes from 200 countries and 7.5 million ticket holders preparing to jam into villages and venues? They better have a Plan B. So far, they don't."— Sally Jenkins, Washington Post

2020/02/26 In a major turning point for the outbreak, WHO Secretary-General, Dr. Tedros Adhanom Ghebreysus reports that the number of new cases outside China exceeded, for the first time since breakout begins, those inside China. The WHO has yet to declare COVID-19 a pandemic, even though it is already present in 48 countries and territories, with more than 81,000 confirmed cases, 3 per cent of them outside China.

2020/02/26 Norway, Romania, Greece, Georgia, Pakistan and North Macedonia detect their first cases of COVID-19.

2020/02/26 CDC Confirms Possible Instance of Community Spread of COVID-19 in U.S.

The Centers for Disease Control and Prevention (CDC) has confirmed an infection with the virus that causes COVID-19 in California in a person who reportedly did not have relevant travel history or exposure to another known patient with COVID-19.

At this time, the patient's exposure is unknown. It's possible this could be an instance of community spread of COVID-19, which would be the first time this has happened in the United States. Community spread means spread of an illness for which the source of infection is unknown. It's also possible, however, that the patient may have been exposed to a returned traveler who was infected.

This case was detected through the U.S. public health system — picked up by astute clinicians. This brings the total number of COVID-19 cases in the United States to 15.

2020/02/26 US-South Korea postpone military training

Republic of Korea (ROK)-US Alliance has postponed combined command post training after the ROK government declared the highest alert level on Covid-19.

2020/02/26 A dog is tested "weak positive" for COVID-19 in Hong Kong. A Pomeranian has tested positive for the coronavirus in Hong Kong. The dog is said to have contracted the virus from its infected owner. The dog did not exhibit any symptoms and tested 'weak positive'. It is currently under quarantine for 14 days. Further reading: https://globalnews.ca/news/6608521/dog-quarantined-coronavirus/

2020/02/27 Estonia, Denmark, Northern Ireland and the Netherlands reported their first coronavirus cases.

2020/02/27 Instead of closing down public sites, a measure that public-health experts have taken in other countries, the head of the shrine in Qom called on pilgrims to keep coming. Cases traced back to Iran have been reported in Azerbaijan, Afghanistan, Bahrain, Canada, Georgia, Iraq, Kuwait, Lebanon, Oman, Pakistan, and the United Arab Emirates. Many of these cases have been linked specifically to visits to Qom.

2020/02/27 Saudi Arabia bans foreign pilgrims from visiting Mecca amid coronavirus fears.

2020/02/27 Japan schools: Prime Minister Shinzo Abe announces that all public schools would close nationwide from March 2 for several weeks.

2020/02/27 Facebook cancels F8 annual developer conference in San Jose, scheduled for May 5–6, due to concerns over the coronavirus.

2020/02/27 Australia says pandemic inevitable. At a press conference, Australia Prime Minister Scott Morrison said that 'the world will soon enter a pandemic phase of the coronavirus.' In an effort to be prepared for the prediction, the country implemented its Emergency Response Plan/coronavirus pandemic preparedness plan. Australia also extended China travel ban to 7 March.

2020/02/27 Chinese city offers $1,400 to people who self-report. Qianjiang in Hubei Province has announced 10,000 yuan ($1,425.96) reward for people with Covid-19 symptoms who report themselves to the authorities. The reward will be provided to confirmed cases.

2020/02/27 Japanese woman tests positive for second time. A Japanese woman from Osaka has tested positive for the coronavirus for the second time. She first tested positive in late January and recovered on 1 February.

2020/02/27 Estonia, Denmark, Northern Ireland and the Netherlands reported their first coronavirus cases.

2020/02/28 WHO upgrades global risk of coronavirus to very high.

The World Health Organization says there is now a "very high" risk of the coronavirus spreading globally.

2020/02/28 Lithuania and Wales reported their first coronavirus cases, with Netherlands and Georgia reporting their second.

2020/02/28 The stock market ended its worst week since 2008 financial crisis.

2020/02/28 There are 62 confirmed cases in the United States, reported by the CDC. Forty-four are from the Diamond Princess cruise, three evacuated from Wuhan, twelve are travel-related, two are person-to-person infections and 1 may be from "community spread."

2020/02/28 The first case of the coronavirus in sub-Saharan Africa has been confirmed in Nigeria. The patient is an Italian citizen who works in Nigeria and flew into the commercial city of Lagos from Milan on 25 February. Authorities say he is stable with no serious symptoms and is being treated at a hospital in the city. Elsewhere on the continent, Algeria and Egypt have also confirmed cases of the disease.

2020/02/28 Dog tests weak positive for coronavirus in Hong Kong for the second time.

2020/02/29 Four unexplained West Coast cases raise fears in the United States. Officials on the US West Coast have reported three more unexplained coronavirus cases, raising concerns the virus could be spreading within the community. The patients - in California, Oregon and Washington State - have no known connection to a badly hit country.

On Friday health officials in California's Santa Clara County said an older woman with chronic health conditions had been diagnosed with Covid-

19. Officials said she is not known to have travelled to a country badly affected by the virus or been in contact with a person who had.

"This new case indicates that there is evidence of community transmission but the extent is still not clear," said Dr. Sara Cody, director of the Santa Clara County Public Health Department.

Oregon health officials said a school employee in Clackamas County had tested positive for the virus. In Washington State, authorities said another case concerned a high school student in Snohomish County.

Neither had any contact with a known case nor any history of travel to an affected region.

These bring the total of unexplained cases in the country to four, after another such case was reported in California on Tuesday.

2020/02/29 Qatar confirmed the first case in the country.

MARCH 2020

2020/03/01 France's famed Louvre museum, the world's most visited, closed on Sunday (Mar 1) as coronavirus cases mounted across Europe and beyond, with the global death toll nearing 3,000. The Louvre museum remained closed Sunday after staff refused to come to work over coronavirus fears. "We apologize for any inconvenience and will keep you informed as the situation develops," the museum said on its website. France, already confirmed one hundred cases and two deaths.

2020/03/01 NASA satellite images show drastic decline in China pollution due to coronavirus.

Scientists attribute the decrease to the economic slowdown in China due to coronavirus. Factory and business closures for the Lunar New Year could also have contributed to the 'dramatic drop-off.'

Satellite images issued by NASA have shown a dramatic decline in pollution levels across China, which is "at least partly" due to an economic slowdown following the outbreak of the new coronavirus, the space agency said on Sunday. The images show concentrations of nitrogen dioxide, "a noxious gas emitted by motor vehicles, power plants and industrial facilities," according to NASA.

The reduction in NO2 pollution was first apparent near Wuhan, the city at the center of the COVID-19 outbreak in China, according to NASA scientists, but eventually spread across the country.

Millions of Chinese citizens have been quarantined, and cities placed in lockdown since the start of the novel coronavirus outbreak.

"This is the first time I have seen such a dramatic drop-off over such a wide area for a specific event," Fei Liu, an air quality researcher at NASA's Goddard Space Flight Center, said in a press release. He added that he had seen a drop in pollution levels in several countries during the 2008 economic recession, but the decrease had been gradual.

2020/03/03 Hong Kong dog is tested weak positive for the third time. Infection is confirmed, and the alternative explanation of an environmental contamination is definitely discarded.

2020/03/04 World Health Organization says the global COVID-19 Case Fatality Rate is 3.4%, three times higher than seasonal flu. President Trump says live on national TV he thinks the number is overestimated. But the United States had reported nine deaths and 129 confirmed cases. That equals to a 6.9% Case Fatality Rate. The highest Case Fatality Rate worldwide. Even higher than Iran´s, Italy's, and China's. And over twice worldwide Case Fatality Rate announced by the WHO.

2020/03/05 Iran to limit travel between major cities and reports more than 3,500 cases. More than three dozen officials and lawmakers have been infected, including a vice president; an adviser to Iran's supreme leader, Ayatollah Ali Khamenei, has died because of the virus. Iranian media reported that another official, Hossein Sheikholeslam, a prominent diplomat and former ambassador to Syria, also had died of the disease.

Saudi Arabia accused the Iranian authorities of having recklessly spread the disease to the Arab monarchy and other countries.

In a statement through the official Saudi Press Agency, the government said five confirmed Saudi cases of the coronavirus disease, known as Covid-19, were Saudi citizens who had visited Iran surreptitiously with help from Iranian officials, who had not stamped their passports. Saudi Arabia has banned its citizens from travel to Iran.

"This behavior poses a serious public health threat to the international community and undermines international efforts to combat Covid-19, putting many communities around the world at risk," the statement said, referring to the illness caused by the coronavirus.

There was no immediate comment by Iran. Messages left with Iran's United Nations Mission for a response were not returned.

2020/03/05 In Europe confirmed cases passing 5,000 and rising fast. The epidemic in Europe will probably get much worse before it is contained, officials warned, as the number of infections across the continent jumped sharply, from fewer than 4,000 on to well over 5,000, only a day after, and with at least 160 deaths.

In the hardest-hit European countries, the number of cases saw the biggest one-day jumps so far: from 3,089 to 3,858 in Italy; from 262 to 482 in Germany; and from 285 to 423 in France. In Netherlands, infections more than doubled, from 38 to 82.

The death toll in Italy, the source of outbreaks in several other countries, leapt from 107 to 148, the highest figure outside of China.

2020/03/05 In the United States, 14 deaths and 233 confirmed cases (CFR 6%). Thousands of New Yorkers self-quarantined. As of March 5, 2020 1,583 patients had been tested at CDC. This does not include testing being done at state and local public health laboratories, which began this week.

2020/03/05 The World Health Organization (WHO) warned Thursday that a "long list" of countries were not showing "the level of political commitment" needed.

"This is not a drill," WHO chief Tedros Adhanom Ghebreyesus told reporters. "This epidemic is a threat for every country, rich and poor."

2020/03/05 IATA warns Covid-19 will cost airlines up to $113billion in revenue this year, as regional airline Flybe collapses, and experts fear others will follow.

2020/03/06 President Emmanuel Macron of France urged citizens to avoid visiting retirement homes and the elderly "as much as possible. Our absolute priority is to protect people who are most vulnerable to the virus," Mr. Macron said on Friday said after visiting a retirement home in Paris, noting that seniors and people who have other illness were most at risk.

2020/03/06 CDC Flawed Test scandal: (Please read this outstanding full article here: https://www.nytimes.com/2020/03/02/health/coronavirus-testing-cdc.html.) And I quote: "We have been really frustrated, because one of the things that is a hallmark of public health labs is that we are usually 'ready, set, go,' and here we were — 'ready, set, wait'," said Scott Becker, chief executive of the Association of Public Health Laboratories.

Late last week, the Food and Drug Administration broke the logjam, authorizing state and local laboratories to do initial testing on their own. If labs had developed and validated a test, they could use it for diagnosis instead of relying on the C.D.C.'s version or waiting for a replacement.

The move greatly expanded the nation's testing capacity, even as the C.D.C. said it was shipping out new test kits to the states.

By that time, however, the agency had tested just under 500 Americans with suspected infections identified by public health officials in the United States. Other nations have tested patients by tens of thousands. China has probably tested millions.

"How come the South Koreans can do 10,000 tests a day and we can't?" said Ralph Baric, who studies coronaviruses and emerging diseases at University of North Carolina.

"Once you knew you had asymptomatic spread and community spread in China, why is it that the United States of America hasn't created tens of thousands of tests?"

2020/03/06 President Trump on Friday signed an $8.3 billion emergency spending bill to confront the coronavirus outbreak and decided to visit the Centers for Disease Control and Prevention in Atlanta, reversing his decision hours earlier to skip touring the nerve center of the government's response to the health crisis.

2020/03/06 Paris Marathon postponed from April 5 to October 18.

2020/03/06 Stock markets in several European countries dropped in early trading Friday, with Frankfurt and London shedding 3.7 and 3.3%, respectively. Stock markets in Japan, South Korea, Hong Kong, Shanghai and Australia all dropped Friday, as uncertainty continues over the epidemic's long-term effect on international business.

2020/03/06 Over 100,000 confirmed cases of COVID-19 worldwide.

2020/03/06 Hubei, the Chinese province at the center of the coronavirus outbreak, reported on Friday that there were no new infections outside its capital, Wuhan. The news is a major milestone in the government's all-out campaign to combat an epidemic that has gripped the country since January.

And with this most excellent news we close this timeline. Hope to the World!

CHAPTER TWO
Take Action

Nor specific medication neither vaccine for COVID-19

About medications: According to the WHO (World Health Organization), "To date, there is no specific medicine recommended to prevent or treat the new coronavirus (2019-nCoV)", and "Antibiotics do not work against viruses, they only work on bacterial infections. COVID-19 is caused by a virus, so antibiotics do not work. Antibiotics should not be used as a means of prevention or treatment of COVID-19. They should only be used as directed by a physician to treat a bacterial infection".

About vaccines: Also according to the WHO," Vaccines against pneumonia, such as pneumococcal vaccine and Haemophilus influenza type B (Hib) vaccine, do not provide protection against the new coronavirus. However, those affected should receive care to relieve symptoms. People with serious illness should be hospitalized. Most patients recover thanks to supportive care.

Possible vaccines and some specific drug treatments are under investigation. They are being tested through clinical trials. WHO is coordinating efforts to develop vaccines and medicines to prevent and treat COVID-19.

The virus is so new and different that it needs its own vaccine. Researchers are trying to develop a vaccine against 2019-nCoV, and WHO is supporting their efforts".

Strengthen your Immune System

Highly recommended further reading:

New Study Shows Only Half of People Infected with Flu Virus Actually Get Sick -- Why? By Dr. Joseph Mercola September 22, 2011

https://articles.mercola.com/sites/articles/archive/2011/09/22/new-study-shows-only-half-of-people-infected-with-flu-virus-actually-get-sick--why.aspx

Best articles from Mercola.com about Immune System support https://search.mercola.com/results.aspx?q=Immune%20system#stq=Immune%20system

You have already read what CDC and WHO have to offer concerning treatment (no specific medications, no vaccines) and prevention (washing your hands, distancing, cleaning surfaces). Not much really!

I think nobody can blame you or me if we try to find something else to help protect ourselves and our loved ones and communities.

Besides all this non pharmaceutical interventions advised by the authorities, which are absolutely correct and most useful, and we all should make part of our everyday life from now on, we feel the need for something more. Something else we can do.

And there are many things we can do.

Note I will share with you only the best advices, from the most reliable sources, and only in case they are absolutely safe and harmless. And you know you should always ask your doctor. And get help as soon as possible if things do no look so well.

These resources are mostly life style options and are intended to ease discomfort. They are useful for any mild viral ailment, like a cold. So they hopefully will help you.

First things first. We, afraid as we are now, info medically infected, imagine that contact with the virus equals infection equals disease. And nothing like that! We have already seen that an unknown number of infected individuals do not develop the disease, they remain asymptomatic. Even during the first month of the epidemic Chinese doctors could somehow discover that a 1.2% of infected patients remained asymptomatic, and an 80.9% developed only mild symptoms. But I have more good news for you! Contact with the virus does not equal disease. In a 2011 study by the University of Michigan, researchers say: "In order to delineate host molecular responses that differentiate symptomatic and asymptomatic Influenza A infection, we inoculated 17 healthy adults with live influenza (H3N2/Wisconsin) and examined changes in host peripheral blood gene expression at 16 time points over 132 hours" (Read full paper here: https://journals.plos.org/plosgenetics/article?id=10.1371/journal.pgen.1002234) Simple said, they inoculated de patients, but only half of them developed symptoms. I mean, all of the subjects were confirmed cases of infection, every one of them developed an immune response to the virus. What was different in the two groups, then? The authors say "Exposure to influenza viruses is necessary, but not sufficient, for healthy human hosts to develop symptomatic illness. The host response is an important determinant of disease progression" So the development of the symptoms of the disease is one kind of immune response to de infection. The asymptomatic group had a different immune response. A much nicer one, I would say.

So, my next question, is there anything I could possible do to develop nicer immune responses? As asymptomatic as possible, please? And the answer is another good news: Yes, there are many things you can do to favor a nicer immune response to a viral infection.

Anything you could and can do to strengthen your immune system. Because, as we have seen before, when we talked about viruses, "Viral infections can cause disease in humans, animals and even plants. However, they are usually eliminated by the immune system, conferring lifetime immunity to the host for that virus. Most viral infections resolve spontaneously in immunocompetent individuals". So the answer to our worries is a new question: How do I become an immunocompetent individual? Or, what is the same, what can I do to strengthen my Immune System?

Think it this way. As Dr., Joseph Mercola so clearly says

"You can greatly lower your risk of coming down with a cold, flu or other illness by modifying your daily lifestyle habits. I haven't missed a day of work due to illness in over 30 years, so I speak from personal experience. I've also seen my health-conscious friends and colleagues enjoy similar benefits. This is clearly not because we have never been exposed to a flu virus … it's a direct result of healthy lifestyle choices.

I like to use the analogy of disease to darkness and health to light. If you shine a light in a dark room it is not dark anymore. Darkness and light simply can't coexist. Similarly, if you are healthy you can have massive exposure to infectious agents and you simply will NOT get sick.

Just like light and darkness, it is very difficult, if not impossible in most cases, for a strong immune system and infectious disease to exist together. It is the state of your immune system -- not the bacteria or virus itself -- that determines whether or not you will get sick, even if you come in contact with the germ." (Article quoted: New Study Shows Only Half of People Infected with Flu Virus Actually Get Sick -- Why? By Dr. Joseph Mercola September 22, 2011 read full article here: https://articles.mercola.com/sites/articles/archive/2011/09/22/new-study-shows-only-half-of-people-infected-with-flu-virus-actually-get-sick--why.aspx

So, which are those almost miraculous daily life habits?

Some of them are the following:

1-**Get enough high quality sleep**;

2-**Avoid exposure to environmental toxins**; (I would add also Quit smoking!)

3-**Optimize Your Vitamin D.** Vitamin D is necessary to activate the immune system. If you are vitamin D deficient you will be at a higher risk of developing lower respiratory tract infections. Best way to increase your vitamin D levels? Enjoy the sun! Get lightly tan. You can get a prescription from your doctor too. You can ask him to check your levels. This is one thing you could do now.

4-**Avoid sugar and fructose and optimize your Leptin and Insulin levels.** Sugar decreases the immune system functioning.

5-Exercise! Exercise improves the circulation of immune cells in your blood. And cuts by half your probability of catching a cold, and by a 30% severity and duration if you sadly catch one.

6-Eat mostly unprocessed food. Prefer raw food. Chemicals present in processed food are toxic and overload your system. Try to avoid them as much as possible.

7-Learn how to deal with stress. You know you are more likely to catch a cold when you are tired or under a lot of stress. Both acute and chronic stress will deteriorate your immune system. Meditate, learn Emotional Freedom Technique, start a Gratitude Journal. Do what you like: exercise, cultivate a hobby, like Gardening or Crafts. Play. Laugh. Get involved in your community. Try to nourish your emotional bonds with family and friends.

Other authors include in this list also **minerals** as magnesium, selenium, zinc, and iodine. Consult your physician. Do not self-medicate.

A paragraph about Vitamin C. There are studies about the use of C vitamin to treat sepsis. Read the following article from Mercola.com: Vitamin C Works for Sepsis. Will It Work for Coronavirus? Analysis by Dr. Joseph Mercola   Fact   Checked https://articles.mercola.com/sites/articles/archive/2020/02/24/iv-vitamin-c.aspx

Recommended further reading:

https://www.newscientist.com/round-up/immune-retune/
https://www.newscientist.com/article/dn21667-immune-retune-eat-yourself-strong/ https://www.newscientist.com/article/dn21672-immune-retune-get-bug-fighting-fit/https://www.newscientist.com/article/dn21671-immune-retune-good-day-sunshine/ https://www.newscientist.com/article/dn21670-immune-retune-safeguard-your-sleep/
https://www.newscientist.com/article/dn21669-immune-retune-dont-stress-out/ https://www.newscientist.com/article/dn21668-immune-retune-befriend-your-bacteria/

How to (correctly) wash your hands

Recommended further reading:

Four of the Most Dangerous Myths About Washing Your Hands https://articles.mercola.com/sites/articles/archive/2011/02/25/myths-about-hand-hygiene.aspx

I know you know how to wash your hands. I thought I knew how to wash my hands. But… As properly washing hands is Rule Number One we should take a minute and check this out. Proper hand washing is a sure and most simple way to kill the pathogens that cause the common cold, Influenza, Pneumonia, Hepatitis A, Acute gastroenteritis, Stomach infections such as salmonella, campylobacter and norovirus and other contagious illnesses and surgical wound complications, including MRSA. (see Dr. Mercola´s article quoted above) Really impressive, don´t you think?

How to wash hands properly: Dr. Mercola explains "It's important to use proper hand washing technique. To make sure you're actually removing the germs when you wash your hands, follow these guidelines:

Use warm water

Use a mild soap

Work up a good lather, all the way up to your wrists, for at least 20 seconds

Make sure you cover all surfaces, including the backs of your hands, wrists, between your fingers, and around and below your fingernails

Rinse thoroughly under running water

Dry your hands with a clean towel or let them air dry

In public places, use a paper towel to open the door as a protection from germs that the handles may harbor

Also remember that your skin is actually your primary defense against bacteria, not the soap, so resist the urge to become obsessive about washing your hands. Over-washing can easily reduce the protective oils in your skin (especially in the winter and dry desert environments) and cause your skin to crack—offering easy entry for bacteria and viruses into your body.

Instead, simply wash your hands when they look dirty, and prior to, or after, performing certain tasks that could spread infection, such as in these instances:

Before and after preparing food, especially when handling raw meat and poultry

Before eating

Before and after treating wounds or taking/giving medicine

Before touching a sick or injured person

Before inserting contact lenses

After using the toilet or changing a diaper

After touching an animal, its toys, leashes, or waste

After blowing your nose or coughing/sneezing into your hands

After handling garbage or potentially contaminated waste

Antibacterial Products Pose Several Health Risks

Once you understand that good-old-fashioned soap and water are just as effective as modern antibacterials, the second issue becomes that of side effects. Traditional soap will not harm your health, other than perhaps dry your skin if used too frequently, whereas antibacterial products like triclosan comes with an array of potentially dangerous side effects."

A paragraph about fever

Recommended further reading:

Do You Make This Common Mistake When Your Child is Sick? By Dr. Joseph Mercola https://articles.mercola.com/sites/articles/archive/2011/02/03/the-benefits-of-fever.aspx

https://www.healthychildren.org/English/health-issues/conditions/fever/pages/Treating-a-Fever-Without-Medicine.aspx

Most virus are temperature sensitive. Most bacteria and viruses actually grow better at temperatures lower than the human body. Fever even impairs their replication. So it makes sense to allow the natural response of the immune system and let body temperature rise.

In their site, **the American Academy of Pediatrics** recommends:

Please read full article at https://www.healthychildren.org/English/health-issues/conditions/fever/pages/Treating-a-Fever-Without-Medicine.aspx

"Treating a Fever Without Medicine

Fevers generally do not need to be treated with medication unless your child is uncomfortable or has a history of febrile convulsions. The fever may be important in helping your child fight the infection.

Even higher temperatures are not in themselves dangerous or significant unless your child has a history of seizures or a chronic disease. Even if your child has a history of a fever-related convulsion and you treat the fever with medication, they may still have this kind of seizure. It is more important to watch how your child is behaving.

If he is eating and sleeping well and has periods of playfulness, he probably doesn't need any treatment. You should also talk with your pediatrician about when to treat your child's fever.

Treatment Suggestions for Fever

Keep your child's room and your home comfortably cool, and dress him lightly. Encourage him to drink extra fluid or other liquids (water, diluted fruit juices, commercially prepared oral electrolyte solutions, gelatin [Jell-O], Popsicles, etc.).

If the room is warm or stuffy, place a fan nearby to keep cool air moving.

Your child does not have to stay in his room or in bed when he has a fever. He can be up and about the house, but should not run around and overexert himself.

If the fever is a symptom of a highly contagious disease (e.g., chickenpox or the flu), keep your child away from other children, elderly people, or people who may not be able to fight infection well, such as those with cancer.

Sponging

In most cases, using oral acetaminophen or ibuprofen is the most convenient way to make your feverish child more comfortable. However, sometimes you may want to combine this with tepid sponging, or just use sponging alone.

Sponging is preferred over acetaminophen or ibuprofen if:

Your child is known to be allergic to, or is unable to tolerate, antipyretic (anti-fever) drugs (a rare case).

It is advisable to combine sponging with acetaminophen or ibuprofen if:

Fever is making your child extremely uncomfortable.

He is vomiting and may not be able to keep the medication in his stomach.

To sponge your child, place him in his regular bath (tub or baby bath), but put only 1 to 2 inches of tepid water (85–90 degrees Fahrenheit, or 29.4–32.2 degrees Celsius) in the basin. If you do not have a bath thermometer, test the water with the back of your hand or wrist. It should feel just slightly warm. Do not use cold water, since that will be uncomfortable and may cause shivering, which can raise his temperature. If your child starts to shiver, then the water is too cold. Shivering can make a fever worse; take your child out of the bath if he shivers.

Seat your child in the water—it is more comfortable than lying down. Then, using a clean washcloth or sponge, spread a film of water over his trunk, arms, and legs. The water will evaporate and cool the body. Keep the room at about 75 degrees Fahrenheit (23.9 degrees Celsius), and continue sponging him until his temperature has reached an acceptable level. Never put rubbing alcohol in the water; it can be absorbed into the skin or inhaled, which can cause serious problems, such as coma.

Usually sponging will bring down the fever by one to two degrees in thirty to forty-five minutes. However, if your child is resisting actively, stop and let him just sit and play in the water. If being in the tub makes him more upset and uncomfortable, it is best to take him out even if his fever is unchanged. Remember, a fever less than 105 degrees Fahrenheit (40.5 degrees Celsius) is in itself not harmful. Last Updated 11/21/2015"

Old Wives Tales

These old fashioned foods proved useful generation after generation. We forgot them, but they are coming back. Some foods really help easing discomfort. Include the necessary ingredients in your next grocery list. Try these recipes. Enjoy them with family and friends.

Bone Broth

Recommended further reading:

Selection of articles about Bone Broth
https://search.mercola.com/results.aspx?q=bone%20broth#stq=bone%20broth

https://recipes.mercola.com/mineral-chicken-broth-recipe.aspx

https://recipes.mercola.com/immune-boosting-vegetable-soup-recipe.aspx

https://recipes.mercola.com/bone-broth-recipe.aspx

Benefits of bone broth:

the gelatin found in bone broth supports proper digestion

Bone broth reduces joint pain and inflammation

Has anti-inflammatory effects

Bone broth contains high amounts of calcium, magnesium, and other nutrients that play an important role in healthy bone formation

Bone broth can be made from any type of bones you like – chicken, beef, pork, or even fish – but seek bones from organically raised, pastured, or grass-fed animals

Bone broth is quite possibly the best food for ill or convalescent people.

An makes you feel good!

How to make your homemade bone broth

(find full recipe here: https://recipes.mercola.com/bone-broth-recipe.aspx)?

Bone Broth Recipe

Calories: 379 per serving Prep Time: 10 minutes Cook Time: 25 minutes
Total Time: 35 minutes Serving Size: 3 quarts
Ingredients

3-4 pounds' beef marrow and knuckle bones

2 pounds' meaty bones such as short ribs

1/2 cup raw apple cider vinegar

4 quarts filtered water

3 celery stalks, halved

3 carrots, halved

3 onions, quartered

Handful of fresh parsley

Sea salt

Procedure

Place bones in a pot or a crockpot, add apple cider vinegar and water, and let the mixture sit for 1 hour so the vinegar can leach the mineral out of the bones.

Add more water if needed to cover the bones.

Add the vegetables bring to a boil and skim the scum from the top and discard.

Reduce to a low simmer, cover, and cook for 24-72 hours (if you're not comfortable leaving the pot to simmer overnight, turn off the heat and let it sit overnight, then turn it back on and let simmer all day the next day)

During the last 10 minutes of cooking, throw in a handful of fresh parsley for added flavor and minerals.

Let the broth cool and strain it, making sure all marrow is knocked out of the marrow bones and into the broth.

Add sea salt to taste and drink the broth as is or store in fridge up to 5 to

7 days or freezer up to 6 months for use in soups or stews.

Would you like to give an extra immune system boost to this broth?

Add some shiitake mushrooms, some hijiki and kombu algae, miso, curcuma and ginger powdered or sliced, cayenne pepper and chia seeds.

Spicy foods are traditionally used in Chinese medicine to support the lungs. And western medicine confirmed their healthy properties. I love spicy foods, especially in winter. I feel they help ease my nose and chest congestion, such as **herbal teas**. My favorite herbal tea for colds? Ginger, curcuma and cinnamon tea, with a big dash of cayenne pepper and some honey. I do not specify amounts because you should better try and find the perfect proportions for your taste. Just simmer in a closed pot and enjoy. When I feel congested I prepare a quart, put it in a thermos, and drink cup after cup. It really works!

Most people, including many physicians, do not realize that 80 percent of your immune system is located in your digestive tract, making a healthy gut a major focal point if you want to achieve optimal health. To support your immune system, you can (and should) include some homemade probiotics like water kefir (my favorite), milk kefir, yogurt, sauerkraut, kimchi and lacto fermented pickles. Why homemade? Because homemade ferments are not pasteurized. You need some of these microorganisms alive to improve your gut flora microbiome. As Dr. Mercola says "Host-specific beneficial bacteria appear to be critical for a healthy immune system, researchers say. The results may increase understanding of the health consequences of highly processed diets, excessive use of antibiotics, and our modern-day obsession with antibacterial cleansers, as absence of the "right" gut microbes can shift the balance toward disease" (Please read full article here: Viruses Worldwide Battled by Gut Microbes
https://articles.mercola.com/sites/articles/archive/2012/07/14/gut-microbes-for-healthy-immune-system.aspx)

Highly recommended further reading:

About spicy food
Why Is Spicy Food Good for You?

https://articles.mercola.com/sites/articles/archive/2015/07/27/spicy-food-benefits.aspx3 Reasons You Should Eat More Spicy Food https://articles.mercola.com/sites/articles/archive/2014/09/27/why-eat-spicy-food.aspx Chili Peppers Could Slow Progression of Lung Metastasis https://articles.mercola.com/sites/articles/archive/2019/04/27/health-benefits-of-chili-peppers.aspx

About homemade ferments

Learn How to Make Cultured Veggies at Home to Boost Your Immune System https://articles.mercola.com/sites/articles/archive/2013/06/01/fermented-vegetables.aspx

Benefits of Homemade Yogurt Versus Commercial https://articles.mercola.com/sites/articles/archive/2017/02/27/homemade-yogurt-benefits.aspx

Fermented Foods: How to 'Culture' Your Way to Optimal Health https://articles.mercola.com/fermented-foods.aspx

About gut flora microbiome and Immune System

Viruses Worldwide Battled by Gut Microbes
https://articles.mercola.com/sites/articles/archive/2012/07/14/gut-microbes-for-healthy-immune-system.aspx)

Gut Microbiome May Be a Game-Changer for Cancer Prevention and Treatment https://articles.mercola.com/sites/articles/archive/2018/06/11/gut-microbiome-game-changer.aspx

Gut Bacteria a Key to Health
https://articles.mercola.com/sites/articles/archive/2017/10/02/optimized-gut-health-benefits.aspx

APPENDIX I

WHO recommendations

The following are the basic protective measures recommended by the World Health Organization

https://www.who.int/emergencies/diseases/novel-coronavirus-2019/advice-for-public

Coronavirus disease (COVID-19) advice for the public

Basic protective measures against the new coronavirus

Stay aware of the latest information on the COVID-19 outbreak, available on the WHO website and through your national and local public health authority. COVID-19 is still affecting mostly people in China with some outbreaks in other countries. Most people who become infected experience mild illness and recover, but it can be more severe for others. Take care of your health and protect others by doing the following:

Wash your hands frequently

Regularly and thoroughly clean your hands with an alcohol-based hand rub or wash them with soap and water.

Why? Washing your hands with soap and water or using alcohol-based hand rub kills viruses that may be on your hands.

Maintain social distancing

Maintain at least 1 meter (3 feet) distance between yourself and anyone who is coughing or sneezing.

Why? When someone coughs or sneezes they spray small liquid droplets from their nose or mouth which may contain virus. If you are too close, you can breathe in the droplets, including the COVID-19 virus if the person coughing has the disease.

Avoid touching eyes, nose and mouth

Why? Hands touch many surfaces and can pick up viruses. Once contaminated, hands can transfer the virus to your eyes, nose or mouth. From there, the virus can enter your body and can make you sick.

Practice respiratory hygiene

Make sure you, and the people around you, follow good respiratory hygiene. This means covering your mouth and nose with your bent elbow or tissue when you cough or sneeze. Then dispose of the used tissue immediately.

Why? Droplets spread virus. By following good respiratory hygiene you protect the people around you from viruses such as cold, flu and COVID-19.

If you have fever, cough and difficulty breathing, seek medical care early

Stay home if you feel unwell. If you have a fever, cough and difficulty breathing, seek medical attention and call in advance. Follow the directions of your local health authority.

Why? National and local authorities will have the most up to date information on the situation in your area. Calling in advance will allow your health care provider to quickly direct you to the right health facility. This will also protect you and help prevent spread of viruses and other infections.

Stay informed and follow advice given by your healthcare provider

Stay informed on the latest developments about COVID-19. Follow advice given by your healthcare provider, your national and local public health authority or your employer on how to protect yourself and others from COVID-19.

Why? National and local authorities will have the most up to date information on whether COVID-19 is spreading in your area. They are best placed to advise on what people in your area should be doing to protect themselves.

Protection measures for persons who are in or have recently visited (past 14 days) areas where COVID-19 is spreading

Follow the guidance outlined above.

Stay at home if you begin to feel unwell, even with mild symptoms such as headache and slight runny nose, until you recover. Why? Avoiding contact with others and visits to medical facilities will allow these facilities to operate more effectively and help protect you and others from possible COVID-19 and other viruses.

If you develop fever, cough and difficulty breathing, seek medical advice promptly as this may be due to a respiratory infection or other serious condition. Call in advance and tell your provider of any recent travel or contact with travelers. Why? Calling in advance will allow your health care provider to quickly direct you to the right health facility. This will also help to prevent possible spread of COVID-19 and other viruses.

When and how to use masks

When to use a mask

If you are healthy, you only need to wear a mask if you are taking care of a person with suspected 2019-nCoV infection.

Wear a mask if you are coughing or sneezing.

Masks are effective only when used in combination with frequent hand-cleaning with alcohol-based hand rub or soap and water.

If you wear a mask, then you must know how to use it and dispose of it properly.

How to put on, use, take off and dispose of a mask

Before putting on a mask, clean hands with alcohol-based hand rub or soap and water.

Cover mouth and nose with mask and make sure there are no gaps between your face and the mask.

Avoid touching the mask while using it; if you do, clean your hands with alcohol-based hand rub or soap and water.

Replace the mask with a new one as soon as it is damp and do not re-use single-use masks.

To remove the mask: remove it from behind (do not touch the front of mask); discard immediately in a closed bin; clean hands with alcohol-based hand rub or soap and water.

Myth busters

Are hand dryers effective in killing the new coronavirus?

No. Hand dryers are not effective in killing the 2019-nCoV. To protect yourself against the new coronavirus, you should frequently clean your hands with an alcohol-based hand rub or wash them with soap and water. Once your hands are cleaned, you should dry them thoroughly by using paper towels or a warm air dryer.

Can an ultraviolet disinfection lamp kill the new coronavirus?

UV lamps should not be used to sterilize hands or other areas of skin as UV radiation can cause skin irritation.

How effective are thermal scanners in detecting people infected with the new coronavirus?

Thermal scanners are effective in detecting people who have developed a fever (i.e. have a higher than normal body temperature) because of infection with the new coronavirus.

However, they cannot detect people who are infected but are not yet sick with fever. This is because it takes between 2 and 10 days before people who are infected become sick and develop a fever.

Can spraying alcohol or chlorine all over your body kill the new coronavirus?

No. Spraying alcohol or chlorine all over your body will not kill viruses that have already entered your body. Spraying such substances can be harmful to clothes or mucous membranes (i.e. eyes, mouth). Be aware that both alcohol and chlorine can be useful to disinfect surfaces, but they need to be used under appropriate recommendations.

Is it safe to receive a letter or a package from China?

Yes, it is safe. People receiving packages from China are not at risk of contracting the new coronavirus. From previous analysis, we know coronaviruses do not survive long on objects, such as letters or packages.

Can pets at home spread the new coronavirus (2019-nCoV)?

At present, there is no evidence that companion animals/pets such as dogs or cats can be infected with the new coronavirus. However, it is always a good idea to wash your hands with soap and water after contact with pets. This protects you against various common bacteria such as E.coli and Salmonella that can pass between pets and humans.

Do vaccines against pneumonia protect you against the new coronavirus?

No. Vaccines against pneumonia, such as pneumococcal vaccine and Haemophilus influenza type B (Hib) vaccine, do not provide protection against the new coronavirus.

The virus is so new and different that it needs its own vaccine. Researchers are trying to develop a vaccine against 2019-nCoV, and WHO is supporting their efforts.

Although these vaccines are not effective against 2019-nCoV, vaccination against respiratory illnesses is highly recommended to protect your health.

Can regularly rinsing your nose with saline help prevent infection with the new coronavirus?

No. There is no evidence that regularly rinsing the nose with saline has protected people from infection with the new coronavirus.

There is some limited evidence that regularly rinsing nose with saline can help people recover more quickly from the common cold. However, regularly rinsing the nose has not been shown to prevent respiratory infections.

Can eating garlic help prevent infection with the new coronavirus?

Garlic is a healthy food that may have some antimicrobial properties. However, there is no evidence from the current outbreak that eating garlic has protected people from the new coronavirus.

Does putting on sesame oil block the new coronavirus from entering the body?

No. Sesame oil does not kill the new coronavirus. There are some chemical disinfectants that can kill the 2019-nCoV on surfaces. These include bleach/chlorine-based disinfectants, either solvents, 75% ethanol, per acetic acid and chloroform.

However, they have little or no impact on the virus if you put them on the skin or under your nose. It can even be dangerous to put these chemicals on your skin.

Does the new coronavirus affect older people, or are younger people also susceptible?

People of all ages can be infected by the new coronavirus (2019-nCoV). Older people, and people with pre-existing medical conditions (such as asthma, diabetes, heart disease) appear to be more vulnerable to becoming severely ill with the virus.

WHO advises people of all ages to take steps to protect themselves from the virus, for example by following good hand hygiene and good respiratory hygiene.

Are antibiotics effective in preventing and treating the new coronavirus?

No, antibiotics do not work against viruses, only bacteria.

The new coronavirus (2019-nCoV) is a virus and, therefore, antibiotics should not be used as a means of prevention or treatment.

However, if you are hospitalized for the 2019-nCoV, you may receive antibiotics because bacterial co-infection is possible.

Are there any specific medicines to prevent or treat the new coronavirus?

To date, there is no specific medicine recommended to prevent or treat the new coronavirus (2019-nCoV).

However, those infected with the virus should receive appropriate care to relieve and treat symptoms, and those with severe illness should receive optimized supportive care. Some specific treatments are under investigation, and will be tested through clinical trials. WHO is helping to accelerate research and development efforts with a range or partners.

WHO World Health Organization recommendations for workplaces' preparedness

Getting your workplace ready for COVID-19

In January 2020 the World Health Organization (WHO) declared the outbreak of a new coronavirus disease in Hubei Province, China to be a Public Health Emergency of International Concern. WHO stated there is a high risk of the 2019 coronavirus disease (COVID-19) spreading to other countries around the world. WHO and public health authorities around the world are taking action to contain the COVID-19 outbreak. However, long term success cannot be taken for granted. All sections of our society – including businesses and employers – must play a role if we are to stop the spread of this disease.

How COVID-19 spreads

When someone who has COVID-19 coughs or exhales they release droplets of infected fluid. Most of these droplets fall on nearby surfaces and objects - such as desks, tables or telephones. People could catch COVID-19 by touching contaminated surfaces or objects – and then touching their eyes, nose or mouth. If they are standing within one meter of a person with

COVID-19 they can catch it by breathing in droplets coughed out or exhaled by them. In other words, COVID-19 spreads in a similar way to flu.

Most persons infected with COVID-19 experience mild symptoms and recover. However, some go on to experience more serious illness and may require hospital care. Risk of serious illness rises with age: people over 40 seem to be more vulnerable than those under 40. People with weakened immune systems and people with conditions such as diabetes, heart and lung disease are also more vulnerable to serious illness.

Simple ways to prevent the spread of COVID-19 in your workplace

The low-cost measures below will help prevent the spread of infections in your workplace, such as colds, flu and stomach bugs, and protect your customers, contractors and employees. Employers should start doing these things now, even if COVID-19 has not arrived in the communities where they operate. They can already reduce working days lost due to illness and stop or slow the spread of COVID-19 if it arrives at one of your workplaces.

• Make sure your workplaces are clean and hygienic

o Surfaces (e.g. desks and tables) and objects (e.g. telephones, keyboards) need to be wiped with disinfectant regularly

o Why? Because contamination on surfaces touched by employees and customers is one of the main ways that COVID-19 spreads

• Promote regular and thorough hand-washing by employees, contractors and customers

o Put sanitizing hand rub dispensers in prominent places around the workplace. Make sure these dispensers are regularly refilled

o Display posters promoting hand-washing – ask your local public health authority for these or look on www.WHO.int.

o Combine this with other communication measures such as offering guidance from occupational health and safety officers, briefings at meetings and information on the intranet to promote hand-washing

o Make sure that staff, contractors and customers have access to places where they can wash their hands with soap and water

o Why? Because washing kills the virus on your hands and prevents the spread of COVID19

• Promote good respiratory hygiene in the workplace

o Display posters promoting respiratory hygiene. Combine this with other communication measures such as offering guidance from occupational health and safety officers, briefing at meetings and information on the intranet etc.

o Ensure that face masks (Ordinary surgical face masks rather than N95 face masks) and / or paper tissues are available at your workplaces, for those who develop a runny nose or cough at work, along with closed bins for hygienically disposing of them

o Why? Because good respiratory hygiene prevents the spread of COVID-19

• Advise employees and contractors to consult national travel advice before going on business trips.

• Brief your employees, contractors and customers that if COVID-19 starts spreading in your community anyone with even a mild cough or low-grade fever (37.3 C or more) needs to stay at home. They should also stay home (or work from home) if they have had to take simple medications, such as paracetamol/acetaminophen, ibuprofen or aspirin, which may mask symptoms of the disease.

o Keep communicating and promoting the message that people need to stay at home even if they have just mild symptoms of COVID-19.

o Display posters with this message in your workplaces. Combine this with other communication channels commonly used in your organization or business.

o Your occupational health services, local public health authority or other partners may have developed campaign materials to promote this message

o Make clear to employees that they will be able to count this time off as sick leave. Things to consider when you and your employees travel

• Before traveling

o Make sure your organization and its employees have the latest information on areas where COVID-19 is spreading. You can find this at https://www.who.int/emergencies/diseases/novel-coronavirus-2019/situation-reports/

o Based on the latest information, your organization should assess the benefits and risks related to upcoming travel plans.

o Avoid sending employees who may be at higher risk of serious illness (e.g. older employees and those with medical conditions such as diabetes, heart and lung disease) to areas where COVID-19 is spreading.

o Make sure all persons travelling to locations reporting COVID-19 are briefed by a qualified professional (e.g. staff health services, health care provider or local public health partner)

o Consider issuing employees who are about to travel with small bottles (under 100 CL) of alcohol-based hand rub. This can facilitate regular hand-washing.

• While traveling:

o Encourage employees to wash their hands regularly and stay at least one meter away from people who are coughing or sneezing

o Ensure employees know what to do and who to contact if they feel ill while traveling.

o Ensure that your employees comply with instructions from local authorities where they are traveling. If, for example, they are told by local authorities not to go somewhere they should comply with this. Your employees should comply with any local restrictions on travel, movement or large gatherings.

• When you or your employees return from traveling:

o Employees who have returned from an area where COVID-19 is spreading should monitor themselves for symptoms for 14 days and take their temperature twice a day.

o If they develop even a mild cough or low grade fever (i.e. a temperature of 37.3 C or more) they should stay at home and self-isolate. This means avoiding close contact (one meter or nearer) with other people, including family members. They should also telephone their healthcare provider or the local public health department, giving them details of their recent travel and symptoms. Getting your business ready in case COVID-19 arrives in your community

• Develop a plan of what to do if someone becomes ill with suspected COVID-19 at one of your workplaces

o The plan should cover putting the ill person in a room or area where they are isolated from others in the workplace, limiting the number of people who have contact with the sick person and contacting the local health authorities.

o Consider how to identify persons who may be at risk, and support them, without inviting stigma and discrimination into your workplace. This could include persons who have recently travelled to an area reporting cases, or other personnel who have conditions that put them at higher risk of serious illness (e.g. diabetes, heart and lung disease, older age).

o Tell your local public health authority you are developing the plan and seek their input.

• Promote regular teleworking across your organization. If there is an outbreak of COVID-19 in your community, the health authorities may advise people to avoid public transport and crowded places. Teleworking will help your business keep operating while your employees stay safe.

• Develop a contingency and business continuity plan for an outbreak in the communities where your business operates

o The plan will help prepare your organization for the possibility of an outbreak of COVID19 in its workplaces or community. It may also be valid for other health emergencies

o The plan should address how to keep your business running even if a significant number of employees, contractors and suppliers cannot come to your place of business - either due to local restrictions on travel or because they are ill.

o Communicate to your employees and contractors about the plan and make sure they are aware of what they need to do – or not do – under the plan. Emphasize key points such as the importance of staying away from work even if they have only mild symptoms or have had to take simple medications (e.g. paracetamol, ibuprofen) which may mask the symptoms

o Be sure your plan addresses the mental health and social consequences of a case of COVID-19 in the workplace or in the community and offer information and support.

o For small and medium-sized businesses without in-house staff health and welfare support, develop partnerships and plans with your local health and social service providers in advance of any emergency.

o Your local or national public health authority may be able to offer support and guidance in developing your plan. Remember: Now is the time to prepare for COVID-19. Simple precautions and planning can make a big difference. Action now will help protect your employees and your business.

WHO recommendations to reduce risk of transmission of emerging pathogens from animals to humans in live animal markets:

On 31 December 2019, WHO was informed of cases of pneumonia of unknown etiology (unknown cause) detected in Wuhan City, Hubei Province of China. A novel coronavirus (2019-nCoV) was identified as the causative virus by Chinese authorities on 7 January.

Investigations are ongoing to evaluate the source of the outbreak, mode(s) of transmission and the extent of infection. Available evidence on the 2019-nCoV virus and previous experience with other coronavirus (MERS-CoV and SARS-CoV) and other respiratory viruses (e.g., avian influenza) suggest that there may be zoonotic transmission associated with the 2019-nCoV.

In light of available evidence and past experience, WHO makes the following general recommendations:

As a general precaution, anyone visiting live animal markets, wet markets or animal product markets, should practice general hygiene measures, including regular hand washing with soap and potable water after touching animals and animal products, avoiding touching eyes, nose or mouth with hands, and avoiding contact with sick animals or spoiled animal products. Any contact with other animals possibly living in the market (e.g., stray cats and dogs, rodents, birds, bats) should be strictly avoided. Attention should also be taken to avoid contact with potentially contaminated animal waste or fluids on the soil or structures of shops and market facilities

The consumption of raw or undercooked animal products should be avoided. Raw meat, milk or animal organs should be handled with care, to avoid cross-contamination with uncooked foods, as per good food safety practices.

Recommendations for at-risk groups

Until more is understood about the 2019-nCoV, people with underlying medical conditions are considered at higher risk of severe disease. Therefore, individuals with these underlying medical conditions should avoid contact with live animal markets, stray animals and wild animals, should not eat animal raw meat. Such recommendations should also be disseminated to travellers and tourists with underlying medical conditions.

Slaughterhouse workers, veterinarians in charge of animal and food inspection in markets, market workers, and those handling live animals and animal products should practice good personal hygiene, including frequent hand washing after touching animals and animal products. They should consider wearing protective gowns, gloves, masks while professionally handling animals and fresh animal products. Equipment and working stations should be disinfected frequently, at least once a day. Protective clothing should be removed after work and washed daily. Workers should avoid exposing family members to soiled work clothing, shoes, or other items that may have come into contact with potentially contaminated material. It is therefore recommended that protective clothes and items remain at the workplace for daily washing.

Based on available information, it is not known if the 2019-nCoV has any impact on the health of animals and no particular event has been reported in any species. As a general recommendation, sick animals should never be slaughtered for consumption; dead animals should be safely buried or destroyed and contact with their body fluids should be avoided without protective clothes. Veterinarians should maintain a high level of vigilance and report any unusual event detected in any animal species present in the markets to veterinary authorities.

APPENDIX II
USA CDC Recommendations

Read full text on https://www.cdc.gov/coronavirus/2019-ncov/about/prevention-treatment.html

There is currently no vaccine to prevent coronavirus disease 2019 (COVID-19). The best way to prevent illness is to avoid being exposed to this virus. However, as a reminder, CDC always recommends everyday preventive actions to help prevent the spread of respiratory diseases, including:

Avoid close contact with people who are sick.

Avoid touching your eyes, nose, and mouth.

Stay home when you are sick.

Cover your cough or sneeze with a tissue, then throw the tissue in the trash.

Clean and disinfect frequently touched objects and surfaces using a regular household cleaning spray or wipe.

Follow CDC's recommendations for using a facemask.

CDC does not recommend that people who are well wear a facemask to protect themselves from respiratory diseases, including COVID-19.

Facemasks should be used by people who show symptoms of COVID-19 to help prevent the spread of the disease to others. The use of facemasks is also crucial for health workers and people who are taking care of someone in close settings (at home or in a health care facility).

Wash your hands often with soap and water for at least 20 seconds, especially after going to the bathroom; before eating; and after blowing your nose, coughing, or sneezing.

If soap and water are not readily available, use an alcohol-based hand sanitizer with at least 60% alcohol. Always wash hands with soap and water if hands are visibly dirty.

Steps to help prevent the spread of COVID-19 if you are sick

https://www.cdc.gov/coronavirus/2019-ncov/about/steps-when-sick.html

If you are sick with COVID-19 or suspect you are infected with the virus that causes COVID-19, follow the steps below to help prevent the disease from spreading to people in your home and community.

Stay home except to get medical care

You should restrict activities outside your home, except for getting medical care. Do not go to work, school, or public areas. Avoid using public transportation, ride-sharing, or taxis.

Separate yourself from other people and animals in your home

People: As much as possible, you should stay in a specific room and away from other people in your home. Also, you should use a separate bathroom, if available.

Animals: You should restrict contact with pets and other animals while you are sick with COVID-19, just like you would around other people. Although there have not been reports of pets or other animals becoming sick with COVID-19, it is still recommended that people sick with COVID-19 limit contact with animals until more information is known about the virus. When possible, have another member of your household care for your animals while you are sick. If you are sick with COVID-19, avoid contact with your pet, including petting, snuggling, being kissed or licked, and sharing food. If you must care for your pet or be around animals while you are sick, wash your hands before and after you interact with pets and wear a facemask. See COVID-19 and Animals for more information.

Call ahead before visiting your doctor

If you have a medical appointment, call the healthcare provider and tell them that you have or may have COVID-19. This will help the healthcare provider's office take steps to keep other people from getting infected or exposed.

Wear a facemask

You should wear a facemask when you are around other people (e.g., sharing a room or vehicle) or pets and before you enter a healthcare provider's office. If you are not able to wear a facemask (for example, because it causes trouble breathing), then people who live with you should not stay in the same room with you, or they should wear a facemask if they enter your room.

Cover your coughs and sneezes

Cover your mouth and nose with a tissue when you cough or sneeze. Throw used tissues in a lined trash can; immediately wash your hands with soap and water for at least 20 seconds or clean your hands with an alcohol-based hand sanitizer that contains 60 to 95% alcohol, covering all surfaces of your hands and rubbing them together until they feel dry. Soap and water should be used preferentially if hands are visibly dirty.

Clean your hands often

Wash your hands often with soap and water for at least 20 seconds or clean your hands with an alcohol-based hand sanitizer that contains 60 to 95% alcohol, covering all surfaces of your hands and rubbing them together until they feel dry. Soap and water should be used preferentially if hands are visibly dirty. Avoid touching your eyes, nose, and mouth with unwashed hands.

Avoid sharing personal household items

You should not share dishes, drinking glasses, cups, eating utensils, towels, or bedding with other people or pets in your home. After using these items, they should be washed thoroughly with soap and water.

Clean all "high-touch" surfaces everyday

High touch surfaces include counters, tabletops, doorknobs, bathroom fixtures, toilets, phones, keyboards, tablets, and bedside tables. Also, clean any surfaces that may have blood, stool, or body fluids on them. Use a household cleaning spray or wipe, according to the label instructions. Labels contain instructions for safe and effective use of the cleaning product including precautions you should take when applying the product, such as wearing gloves and making sure you have good ventilation during use of the product.

Monitor your symptoms

Seek prompt medical attention if your illness is worsening (e.g., difficulty breathing). Before seeking care, call your healthcare provider and tell them that you have, or are being evaluated for, COVID-19. Put on a facemask before you enter the facility. These steps will help the healthcare provider's office to keep other people in the office or waiting room from getting infected or exposed. Ask your healthcare provider to call the local or state health department. Persons who are placed under active monitoring or facilitated self-monitoring should follow instructions provided by their local health department or occupational health professionals, as appropriate.

If you have a medical emergency and need to call 911, notify the dispatch personnel that you have, or are being evaluated for COVID-19. If possible, put on a facemask before emergency medical services arrive.

Discontinuing home isolation

Patients with confirmed COVID-19 should remain under home isolation precautions until the risk of secondary transmission to others is thought to be low. The decision to discontinue home isolation precautions should be made on a case-by-case basis, in consultation with healthcare providers and state and local health departments.

Footnote

Fever may be subjective or confirmed

Close contact is defined as -

a) being within approximately 6 feet (2 meters) of a COVID-19 case for a prolonged period of time; close contact can occur while caring for, living with, visiting, or sharing a health care waiting area or room with a COVID-19 case

– or –

b) having direct contact with infectious secretions of a COVID-19 case (e.g., being coughed on)

If such contact occurs while not wearing recommended personal protective equipment or PPE (e.g., gowns, gloves, NIOSH-certified disposable N95 respirator, eye protection), criteria for PUI consideration are met".

Data to inform the definition of close contact are limited. Considerations when assessing close contact include the duration of exposure (e.g., longer exposure time likely increases exposure risk) and the clinical symptoms of the person with COVID-19 (e.g., coughing likely increases exposure risk as does exposure to a severely ill patient). Special consideration should be given to those exposed in health care settings.

Nonpharmaceutical Interventions (NPIs) Recommended by USCDC:

The following texts explain all Nonpharmaceutical Interventions (NPIs) recommended by the CDC in the event of a flu pandemics. They clearly apply to de COVID-19 epidemics and so are much worth to know and practice in everyday life.

Protect yourself and others from getting and spreading respiratory illnesses like pandemic flu.

https://www.cdc.gov/nonpharmaceutical-interventions/index.html

Nonpharmaceutical Interventions (NPIs) are actions, apart from getting vaccinated and taking medicine, that people and communities can take to help slow the spread of illnesses like pandemic influenza (flu). NPIs are also known as community mitigation strategies. When a new flu virus spreads among people, causing illness worldwide, it is called pandemic flu. Because a pandemic flu virus is new, the human population has little or no immunity against it. This allows the virus to spread quickly from person to person worldwide. NPIs are among the best ways of controlling pandemic flu when vaccines are not yet available.

Nonpharmaceutical Interventions (NPIs) include:

What you can do personally (Personal NPIs): Stay home when you are sick. Cover your coughs and sneezes with a tissue. Wash your hands often with soap and water.

What communities can do (Community NPIs): Implement social distancing interventions in schools, workplaces, and at events.

What everyone can do to keep the environment germ-free (Environmental NPIs): Clean frequently touched surfaces and objects like door knobs.

Personal NPIs: Everyday Preventive Actions

What are personal nonpharmaceutical interventions (NPIs)?

Personal NPIs are everyday preventive actions, apart from pharmaceutical interventions such as getting vaccinated and taking medicine that can help keep yourself and others from getting and spreading respiratory illnesses like the flu. They include:

Staying home when you are sick.

Covering coughs and sneezes with a tissue.

Washing hands with soap and water or using hand sanitizer when soap and water is not available.

During a flu pandemic there are measures you can take in addition to these everyday preventive actions. They include:

Staying home if you have been exposed to a family or household member who is sick.

Covering your nose and mouth with a mask or cloth if you are sick and around people or at a mass gathering in a community where the pandemic is already occurring.

Public health professionals need the help of administrators for schools, workplaces, and community events to prevent the spread of respiratory illnesses like pandemic flu in their area. Educating and reminding people to take these everyday preventive actions consistently at home, at school, at work, and at a gathering is an important part of an organization's or community's strategy for minimizing the risks caused by flu and other respiratory illnesses.

The actions you take and plans you make today matter. To ensure the greatest impact, CDC recommends that communities and organizations incorporate a combination of personal, community, and environmental NPIs into their pandemic flu plans.

Why are personal NPIs important?

The flu virus is believed to spread mainly from person to person through droplets that come from the nose and mouth when a sick person coughs, sneezes, or talks. The flu virus may also spread when people touch something with flu virus on it, and then touch their eyes, nose, or mouth. Many other viruses that cause respiratory illnesses spread this way, too.

While getting an annual flu vaccination is the best way to prevent seasonal flu, personal NPIs are simple everyday preventive actions that people can take to help lower their risk of coming in contact with flu and other similar viruses. These everyday preventive actions serve as an extra layer of protection even after people are vaccinated.

In the event that a new flu virus emerges that can rapidly spread from person to person worldwide, causing a flu pandemic, a vaccine may not be immediately available. During a pandemic, personal NPIs become some of the most important ways that individuals can protect themselves and others from the flu.

Community NPIs: Flu Prevention in Community Settings

What are community nonpharmaceutical interventions (NPIs)?

Community NPIs are policies and strategies, apart from pharmaceutical interventions such as vaccination and medical treatment delivery methods, that organizations and communities put into place to help slow the spread of illness during an infectious disease outbreak, such as pandemic flu. Two of the most commonly used community NPIs include:

Social distancing: Creating ways to increase distance between people in settings where people commonly come into close contact with one another. Specific priority settings include schools, workplaces, events, meetings, and other places where people gather.

Closures: Temporarily closing child care centers, schools, places of worship, sporting events, concerts, festivals, conferences, and other settings where people gather.

Why are community NPIs important?

Annual flu vaccinations are the best way for people to prevent seasonal flu. However, if a new flu virus emerges that can rapidly spread from person to person worldwide, causing a flu pandemic, a vaccine may not be immediately available.

This makes planning and working together even more important for a community. Social distancing and closures interventions, while difficult to plan and carry out, can be the most effective ways that a community can protect itself from a pandemic's negative impact.

The actions you take and plans you make today matter. To ensure the greatest impact, CDC recommends that communities and organizations incorporate a combination of personal, community, and environmental NPIs into their pandemic flu plans.

Community NPIs, like social distancing and closures, require careful planning and coordination. Public health professionals, planners, and leaders need to work together to help reduce the risk to their organizations and community from respiratory illnesses like pandemic flu. Recommendations include:

Connecting. Collaborate with other professionals, leaders, and administrators in different settings to identify challenges and how they can be overcome in your community.

Planning. When planning for social distancing and closures, seek ideas for what has worked well in the past or could be improved next time. By gathering data, you can identify strategies for making these interventions work smoothly and with as little disruption as possible to your organization or community.

Sharing. Communicate what you have tried and the obstacles you have faced so that other organizations and communities can also benefit from the work you have done.

Environmental NPIs: Surface Cleaning

What are environmental nonpharmaceutical interventions (NPIs)?

Environmental NPIs include routine surface cleaning that helps to eliminate the flu virus from frequently touched surfaces and objects, such as toys, refrigerator handles, desks, and door knobs in homes, childcare facilities, schools, workplaces, and other settings where people regularly gather.

Public health professionals need the help of administrators of schools, workplaces, and community events to prevent the spread of respiratory illnesses like pandemic flu in their area. Educating and reminding people to clean frequently touched surfaces and objects consistently at home, at school, at work, and at large gatherings are an important part of an organization's or community's strategy for minimizing the risks caused by flu and other respiratory illnesses.

The actions you take and plans you make today matter. To ensure the greatest impact, CDC recommends that communities and organizations incorporate a combination of personal, community, and environmental NPIs into their pandemic flu plans.

Why are environmental NPIs important?

The flu virus is thought to spread mainly from person to person through droplets that come from the nose and mouth when a sick person coughs, sneezes, or talks. The flu virus also may spread when people touch contaminated surfaces or objects, and then touch their eyes, nose, or mouth. Many other viruses that cause respiratory illnesses spread this way, too.

The flu virus can live and potentially infect other people for up to 48 hours after being left behind on a surface. Although the flu virus can survive on hands for only 3 to 5 minutes, if other people later touch a contaminated surface and then touch their eyes, nose, or mouth, they can be exposed to the flu.

While getting an annual flu vaccination is the best way to prevent seasonal flu, environmental NPIs are simple everyday preventive actions that people take to help lower their risk of coming in contact with flu and other similar viruses on surfaces. Routine surface cleaning acts as an extra layer of protection even after people are vaccinated.

In the event that a new flu virus emerges that can rapidly spread from person to person worldwide, causing a flu pandemic, a vaccine may not be immediately available. During a pandemic, routine surface cleaning becomes an important way that individuals can protect themselves and others from the flu.

Flu Prevention at a Mass Gathering

Flu can spread easily at mass gatherings, such as concerts, festivals, meetings, conferences, places of worship, and sporting events. Those traveling to and from mass gatherings can also spread flu to other communities and to family members when they return home.

Note this text is intended for seasonal flu outbreaks. But this NPI are to be applied in every public place (shopping malls, train, metro and bus stations, etc.) You can download this flyer here: https://www.cdc.gov/nonpharmaceutical-interventions/pdf/protect-yourself-from-flu-public-event-item4.pdf

Protect Yourself from Flu at a Large Public Event

National Center for Emerging and Zoonotic Infectious Diseases

Division of Global Migration and Quarantine

Event attendees:

You can protect your health and the health of others while attending a public event. Flu can spread quickly when lots of people are close together for a long time. Plan to stay home if you're sick. By practicing healthy habits, you will be doing your part to help prevent the spread of flu.

Take these actions to help keep yourself and others well:

Get vaccinated.

Stay home if you're sick.

– Keep your distance (6 feet or more) from others at home or if you have to leave (to visit the doctor's office).

If you have a fever, stay home for at least 24 hours after your fever is gone without using medicine that lowers fever.

Cover your nose and mouth with a tissue when you cough or sneeze.

– Throw away dirty tissues.

Use your sleeve or elbow if you don't have a tissue.

Wash or sanitize your hands afterwards.

Wash your hands often.

– Wash with soap and water for at least 20 seconds (the time it takes to hum the "Happy Birthday" song twice).

Use hand sanitizer with at least 60% alcohol if you don't have soap and water.

Try not to touch surfaces and objects that are used and shared often.

Try to keep your distance from people who are sick.

– Limit actions like shaking hands, hugging, and kissing your fellow event attendees.

APPENDIX III
CDC Recommendations for Pandemic Influenza

Please read carefully the following text. It is intended for a flu pandemic, but the Non Pharmaceutical Interventions described here apply to the current COVID-19 epidemics. You can download the brochure here:

https://www.cdc.gov/nonpharmaceutical-interventions/pdf/gr-pan-flu-npi.pdf

And many other useful printable documents.

Get Your Community Ready for Pandemic Influenza

Suggested citation:

Get Your Community Ready for Pandemic Influenza, 2017. Atlanta, GA: Community Interventions for Infection Control Unit, Division of Global Migration and Quarantine, National Center for Emerging and Zoonotic Infectious Diseases,

Centers for Disease Control and Prevention, April 2017.

Contents

Keep the Public Healthy by Planning for Pandemic Influenza

Influenza, also known as "the flu," is a contagious respiratory illness caused by influenza viruses that infect the nose, throat, and lungs (see flu symptoms and complications). Flu spreads mostly by droplets containing flu viruses traveling through the air (up to 6 feet) when a sick person coughs or sneezes. Less often, people might get flu by touching surfaces or objects with flu viruses on them and then touching their eyes, nose, or mouth. Flu can spread quickly from sick people to others who are in close contact in community settings, such as childcare facilities, schools, workplaces, and large events. Vaccination is the first and best way to prevent flu and potentially serious flu-related complications. CDC recommends a yearly flu vaccine for everyone 6 months and older.

CDC also recommends that people practice everyday preventive actions (or personal NPIs) at all times to protect themselves and their loved ones from flu and other respiratory infections (see Page 5). Millions of people in the United States get sick with the flu each year, and hundreds of thousands of people are hospitalized. These numbers may significantly increase during a flu pandemic. Flu pandemics are much less common but can occur at any time. Just as you prepare for seasonal flu, you should prepare for pandemic flu.

Pandemic flu is not seasonal flu.

A flu pandemic can occur when a novel flu virus becomes capable of efficient and sustained human to-human transmission and then spreads globally. Influenza viruses with pandemic potential include nonhuman viruses (i.e., they are new to humans, though they circulate in animals in parts of the world) so people have little to no immunity against them. Human infections with these viruses have rarely occurred, but if one of these viruses changed in such a way that it could infect humans easily and spread easily from person to person, a flu pandemic could result.

A pandemic could overwhelm normal operations in our most vital community organizations, such as hospitals, schools, public transportation, workplaces, and community-based human services organizations.

Read more about the important differences between seasonal flu and pandemic flu.

Updated community mitigation guidelines can help you plan for pandemic flu.

In April 2017, the Centers for Disease Control and Prevention (CDC) released its Community Mitigation Guidelines to Prevent Pandemic Influenza —United States, 2017. The updated guidelines can assist state, tribal, local, and territorial public health officials with pre-pandemic flu planning. CDC also developed audience-specific pandemic flu NPI planning guides for individuals and households, educational settings, workplace settings, community- and faith-based organizations serving vulnerable populations, and planners of large events.

During a flu pandemic, CDC will work closely with state, tribal, local, and territorial public health officials to protect the public's health. CDC will advise public health officials on the use of NPIs and other pandemic countermeasures (such as vaccines and antivirals) to help slow the spread of disease.

As a public health communicator, you play a key role in flu readiness. Communication is integral to helping communities prevent the spread of pandemic flu. State and local public health departments should have an emergency operations or contingency plan in place that includes provisions for pandemic flu. Ensure that your emergency communication plan includes strategies for promoting the use of NPIs and other flu prevention measures before and during a flu pandemic. Visit CDC's Emergency Preparedness and Response page for more information about emergency planning and communication.

NPIs can help slow the spread of flu.

When a new flu virus emerges, a well-matched pandemic flu vaccine will be the most effective countermeasure to prevent widespread transmission. However, a pandemic flu vaccine may not be readily available during the initial 4-6 months of a pandemic, given current vaccine production technology. Preventing the spread of a pandemic flu virus will be a public health priority. When a vaccine is not available, NPIs are the best way to help slow the spread of flu. They include personal, community, and environmental actions that are more efficient when used together.

Personal NPIs are everyday preventive actions that can help keep people from getting and/ or spreading flu. These actions include staying home when you are sick, covering your coughs and sneezes with a tissue, and washing your hands often with soap and water.

Community NPIs are strategies that organizations and community leaders can use to help limit face-to-face contact. These strategies may include making sick-leave policies more flexible, promoting telework, avoiding close contact with others, and scheduling remote meetings.

Environmental NPIs are surface cleaning measures that remove germs from frequently touched surfaces and objects.

Information provided to the public must be correct, brief, and simply written for diverse audiences. Clear communication helps audiences understand, remember, and use information the first time they read it.

Did you know that an estimated 61 million people in the United States were sick during the 2009 H1N1 flu pandemic? Responding to an influenza pandemic will require an integrated approach that includes both the development of a pandemic flu vaccine and the use of NPIs. Pre-pandemic planning is critical for developing a comprehensive communication plan that clearly explains the importance of both flu vaccination and NPIs in slowing the spread of flu in communities. Your communication plan should provide partners, stakeholders, and the public with information about seasonal and pandemic flu before each flu season and before a flu pandemic.

CDC has developed recommendations for preventing the spread of flu in communities. It is important that communities actively adopt and practice good personal health habits before a flu pandemic occurs. Educate key partners and stakeholders and the public about additional community NPI actions that may be recommended by public health officials, if a flu pandemic occurs. These actions can help keep people healthy.

EVERYDAY PREVENTIVE ACTIONS Everyone should always practice good personal health habits to help prevent flu. Stay home when you are sick. Stay home for at least 24 hours after you no longer have a fever or signs of a fever without the use of fever-reducing medicines. Cover your coughs and sneezes with a tissue. Wash your hands often with soap and water for at least 20 seconds. Use at least a 60% alcohol-based hand sanitizer if soap and water are not available. Clean frequently touched surfaces and objects.

NPIs RESERVED FOR A FLU PANDEMIC Communities should be prepared to take these additional actions if recommended by public health officials. * Stay home if someone in your house is sick. Increase the space to at least 3 feet between people, and limit face-to-face contact in schools, workplaces, and at large events, as much as possible. Temporarily dismiss students attending childcare facilities, K-12 schools, and institutions of higher education. Modify, postpone, or cancel large events. *These additional actions may be recommended for severe, very severe, or extreme flu pandemics.

Anyone can get sick from flu, but some people may be at greater risk than others for serious complications from flu. In your emergency communication plan, identify and connect with organizations that serve vulnerable and high-risk populations. Work with them to plan effective and creative ways to disseminate health messages and materials before and during a flu pandemic

SEASONAL FLU HIGH-RISK POPULATIONS

- Adults 65 years and older
- Pregnant women and women less than 2 weeks postpartum
- Children younger than 5, especially those younger than 2 years' old
- Residents of nursing homes and long-term care facilities
- People with chronic medical conditions, such as asthma, heart

disease, and blood disorders

VULNERABLE POPULATIONS

❑ People who are culturally, geographically, or socially isolated:

❑ People with limited English language skills

❑ Migrant workers, immigrants, and refugees

❑ People who are experiencing homelessness

❑ People with physical disabilities, limitations, or impairments

❑ People with mental illness

❑ People who are in prison, jail, corrections, and immigrant or juvenile detention centers

❑ Low-income people, single-parent families, and residents of public housing

Building community trust is important. Building trust should start before a flu pandemic occurs. It requires understanding the community's needs and concerns about pandemic flu and NPIs. Building awareness and engaging community leaders, organizations, and the public in pandemic flu education and training can help increase their confidence during emergencies.

Before an Influenza Pandemic Occurs: Plan

Did you know preparedness should focus on strengthening the systems and structures that support effective and well-coordinated communication, and not solely on the development of communication messages?

A good emergency communication plan encourages community leaders and stakeholders to plan now for pandemic influenza and other types of emergencies. Before a flu pandemic occurs, focus on raising awareness and educating audiences about NPIs and other public health flu-prevention strategies. Identify key community relationships, and leverage them to help educate and prepare audiences. It takes time to build relationships. Engage internal and external partners and stakeholders early in your planning process. Coordinating your planning efforts with them can help establish strong lines of communication and ensure that information is consistent before and during a pandemic.

Become familiar with key flu prevention messages and NPI recommendations

✔ Read and understand "Everyday Preventive Actions" (Page 5). This list features good personal health habits that protect against flu and other illnesses. Emphasize these habits in your communications every flu season, and especially during a flu pandemic.

✔ Read and understand "NPIs Reserved for a Flu Pandemic" (Page 5). Some protective strategies will only be recommended if the severity of a pandemic is much greater than that for seasonal flu. You should be prepared to communicate this information during a flu pandemic—this is very important.

✔ Read and understand CDC's audience specific pandemic flu NPI planning guides and communication materials. Tailored guides and resources addressing pandemic flu planning are available for individuals and households, educational settings, workplace settings, community- and faith-based organizations serving vulnerable populations, and planners of large events.

✔ Take CDC's NPI 101 Web-based training. State, tribal, local, and territorial public health officials can complete a 90-minute training to increase their understanding of NPIs and how to implement them during a flu pandemic. Access the NPI 101 Training.

Update your existing emergency communication plan

✔ Meet with your existing emergency planning and operations team to update the emergency communication plan for your state or community. Review all aspects of your plan, such as personnel, communication strategies, trainings, tools, policies, equipment, systems and procedures for clearing and approving information, and other resources. Develop or update your plan based on various scenarios your state or community may face during a flu pandemic.

✔ Establish systems for sharing information with key partners and stakeholders. Identify everyone in your chain of communication (e.g., new and existing partners and stakeholders, others in your own agency, and other health departments), and create or update a comprehensive contact list. Maintain up-to-date primary and secondary contact information for everyone in the chain. Determine when and what type of information to share with those in your communication chain. Identify platforms, such as a hotline, automated text messaging, email, social media, and a website, to help disseminate information to internal and external partners and audiences. Help community members prepare for pandemic flu

✔ Create a pandemic flu communication workgroup with representatives from key partners and stakeholders. Include communication, marketing, and public relations professionals who work in various community settings, such as childcare programs, healthcare facilities, pharmacies, schools, workplaces, community- and faith based organizations, and public and private organizations. Discuss with the workgroup the emergency communication plan for your state or community. Determine how to coordinate pandemic flu communication between workgroup members. Encourage their participation in other communitywide flu-readiness activities. Note: Inform workgroup members about workshops, programs, and other activities they can implement within their organizations to inspire the public to consistently practice good personal health habits and prepare for emergencies.

✔ Engage communities in a dialogue about pandemic flu readiness. Conduct needs assessments or focus groups with community members to gather information about their knowledge, attitudes, beliefs, and challenges related to NPIs and pandemic flu. Use their feedback to improve your communication strategies, messages, and materials. Note: Work closely with workgroup members and key partners and stakeholders to address flu readiness challenges and barriers identified by audiences in your community. Identifying solutions to help audiences move past barriers may help people change habits and better adapt to changing circumstances during a pandemic.

✔ Encourage community members to plan for flu. Promote the practice of everyday preventive actions before a pandemic occurs. Identify up-to-date resources and tools to help community members plan and prepare for pandemic flu.

Identify information needs and community resources

✔ Identify target audiences and communication channels. Work with workgroup members and key partners and stakeholders to define audiences and develop strategies to reach every member of the community. Additional strategies may be needed to reach high-risk and vulnerable populations. Address any gaps in communication resources, materials, or processes. Note: Some NPI actions may draw public attention and can have negative psychosocial and economic consequences on groups and individuals to which they are applied during a pandemic, especially to high-risk and vulnerable populations. Include in your communication plan strategies and messages that address fear, stigmatization, and discrimination.

✔ Identify the training needs of workgroup members and key partners and stakeholders. Identify existing trainings or develop new trainings about NPIs, decision-making, and risk communication. Ensure communicators across sectors have the necessary skills and understanding to develop emergency communication plans and promote flu readiness within their organizations.

✔ Become a resource for pandemic flu information. Each flu pandemic is different. Ready-to-use messages and materials, such as fact sheets, checklists, and frequently asked questions, will need to be tailored to the pandemic and to each audience. Prepare resources that educate people about flu terminology (like "flu severity") and the importance of adopting NPI measures (like staying home when sick). Use plain language, and include examples and pictures in your materials to improve understanding. Visit CDC's NPI website for messages and materials about preventing pandemic flu. Visit CDC's Health Literacy page for more information about plain language. Assess procedures and technology resources needed for timely communication during a pandemic

✔ Review, exercise, and update communication policies, procedures, and systems for updating, clearing, approving, and disseminating information (both internally and externally). Make sure information is accurate and consistent during an emergency and flows promptly and frequently to the correct audiences. Review your system for tracking and responding to inquiries received from the public, partners, and stakeholders. Note: Communication after-action reports and improvement plans (AARs/IPs) from recent public health emergency responses can offer practical and helpful insights. Visit CDC's Pandemic Flu page for pandemic flu resources.

✔ Identify existing and needed technology resources. Assess and update the availability of technology and equipment, such as mobile phones, computers, Internet access, and wireless devices, so they are ready for immediate use. If needed resources do not exist inside your organization, create a plan for acquiring them or identify sources from which you can access technology during a flu pandemic.

Plan for the dissemination of flu information

✔ Create a plan for interacting with news media. The media can serve as a vital link in providing up-to-date information and helping to deliver key messages to the public. Develop a strategy for communicating directly with the public, working with the media, and responding to inquiries.

✔ Identify multiple spokespersons or subject matter experts. Experts who will serve as spokespersons should be experienced in public health emergencies and pandemic flu. Include representatives from limited English-speaking communities. Provide training, as needed, so they are comfortable speaking to news media and able to answer challenging questions using plain language (clear communication). See Crisis and Emergency Risk Communication: By Leaders for Leaders to learn more about the role of a spokesperson.

✔ Develop a plan for using current social media. Plan ways to incorporate popular or topical social media platforms that can help you promote key messages and quickly update people with new information. Social media platforms also provide direct access to your target audiences, giving you opportunities to engage in real-time discussions for information gathering and evaluation purposes.

✔ Develop a communication evaluation plan. Use these questions to help you measure the effectiveness of your emergency communication plan:

❑ Can your audiences find, understand, and use your information?

❑ Are your key messages culturally appropriate and in plain language?

❑ Are you successfully increasing awareness by disseminating resources and materials?

❑ Are communication activities being successfully coordinated with internal and external partners and stakeholders?

❑ Can you confirm that timely information is being provided throughout the duration of the pandemic?

❑ Is misinformation being spread on social media, or elsewhere? If so, how are you counteracting it?

✔ Test and update your emergency communication plan every 12–18 months. Practice the actions outlined in your plan. Ensure systems and procedures support communication activities needed during a flu pandemic.

Refine messages, materials, and tools. Encourage workgroup members to test the emergency communication plans for their organizations.

Create short, concise, focused messages with action steps.

Consider creating pandemic flu message maps with internal and external partners that can be quickly used or adapted when needed. Communication should be audience specific, culturally appropriate, clear, concise, and in plain language. Working with partners to develop messages can create a more efficient flow of communication when a pandemic occurs.

During an Influenza Pandemic: Take Action

Did you know that most people are not familiar with the terms NPI and pandemic flu?

Maintain ongoing communication with your workgroup members, partners, and stakeholders once an influenza pandemic is declared. Coordinate pandemic flu communication activities with news media and other channels to ensure consistent messaging. If you must use technical terminology and concepts, be sure to define them and include examples to help improve understanding. For example, create messages that clearly explain pandemic influenza and NPIs. CDC also will regularly send out "key message" documents that provide current and accurate information about the pandemic.

Your communication should be early, empathetic, accurate, and effective. Early communication of flu information helps limit misinformation and rumors that could contribute to confusion and fear. Empathetic communication conveys concern and reassurance, empowers people, and reduces emotional turmoil. Accurate communication provides the facts about a situation and what is being done to resolve it. Effective communication helps build understanding and guide the public, media, healthcare providers, and other groups in responding to pandemic flu and complying with public health recommendations.

Put your emergency communication plan into action

✔ Stay informed about the pandemic. Work closely with CDC to get up-to-date information about flu activity across the United States and how it may affect your state or local community.

✔ Provide instructions for NPI implementation. Explain why NPIs are necessary and effective when implemented early and practiced throughout the pandemic. Give details about what, how, when, and where NPIs will be implemented in the community. Access CDC's updated Community Mitigation Guidelines by visiting http://dx.doi. org/10.15585/mmwr. rr6601a1. See Crisis and Emergency Risk Communication for more information about communicating during an emergency.

✔ Continue to promote the daily practice of everyday preventive actions. Provide frequent updates to the public to ensure they understand their risk for getting and spreading flu and how to reduce their risk. Encourage people to stay home and away from others when they are sick and to practice good health habits.

SAMPLE PANDEMIC FLU MESSAGES FOR THE PUBLIC:

❏ A flu pandemic occurs when a new flu virus, different from seasonal flu viruses, appears and spreads quickly between people worldwide.

❏ Most people are not immune to the pandemic flu virus.

❏ There are actions that people and communities can take, apart from getting vaccinated and taking medicines, to help slow the spread of flu viruses.

❏ Practice everyday preventive actions to help protect yourself and others from getting sick—stay home when you are sick, cover your coughs and sneezes with a tissue, wash your hands often, and clean frequently touched surfaces and objects.

❏ Get a pandemic flu vaccination as soon as it is available in your community.

Communicate frequently with those in your communication chain

✔ Always give simple, credible, accurate, consistent, and timely information. Be transparent and share what is known and unknown about the flu situation in your state or community. Use a variety of communication channels to distribute audience-specific health messages and materials. Provide additional resources and Web links where the public can find reliable NPI and pandemic flu information. See Crisis and Emergency Risk Communication: By Leaders for Leaders to learn more about the role of a spokesperson.

✔ Update everyone in your communication chain regularly. Share updated information with your workgroup members, partners, and stakeholders to help them make decisions.

✔ Communicate flu prevention information to those who are vulnerable and at high risk for flu complications. Work with partners to implement communication strategies for reaching high-risk and vulnerable populations in your community (for example, people who are homeless or have limited English-language skills). See People at High Risk of Developing Flu–Related Complications for a list of who may be at high risk for flu complications. To learn how community- and faith-based organizations can help vulnerable populations during a pandemic, visit https://www.cdc.gov/nonpharmaceutical-interventions/pdf/gr-pan-flucom-faith-org-serv-vul-pop.pdf.

Monitor and evaluate your efforts, and change communications as needed

✔ Monitor all media sources. Use a variety of media channels to address misinformation and gather feedback about the response.

✔ Implement actions outlined in your evaluation plan. Document communication activities that have and have not happened. Include details about why the activities did not occur or about changes made to the emergency communication plan during the pandemic.

Develop strong communication strategies and campaigns. Communication should be transparent, accurate, and engaging. Plan ways to include audiences in the development of messages and materials before a pandemic occurs. Get Your Community Ready for Pandemic Flu.

After an Influenza Pandemic Has Ended: Follow Up

Did you know health communicators can disseminate well-designed information that achieves behavior change?

As influenza activity during a pandemic declines, work with your workgroup members to identify criteria for phasing out and ending flu-prevention communication activities. Implement your evaluation plan to determine the effectiveness of communication activities during the pandemic. Maintain an attitude of preparedness by continuing to collaborate with workgroup members, partners, and stakeholders to enhance their communication skills on flu readiness and other health issues. Use data from the response to identify new communication strategies and campaigns to facilitate long-term behavior change.

Evaluate the effectiveness of your emergency communication plan

✔ Discuss and note lessons learned. Gather feedback from the public, workgroup members, partners, and stakeholders to improve your plan. Discuss which communication channels, materials, tools, and messages were successful, which were unsuccessful, and which were missing from your plan. Determine whether target audiences were reached. Identify any needs you may have for additional resources.

✔ Maintain and expand your pandemic flu communication workgroup. Look for ways to expand community partnerships. Identify trusted representatives from the community and federal, state, or local agencies or organizations needed to help you prepare for pandemic flu, and make an effort to include them in your communication planning activities if they were not previously included.

✔ Update and practice your emergency communication plan every 12–18 months, or as aspects of your agency change. Modify your plan and policies based on lessons learned and on NPI strategies and messaging implemented during the pandemic. Replace necessary communication supplies and equipment.

Congratulations on planning for a flu pandemic

A flu pandemic can occur at any time, and you can make a big difference by having your emergency communication plan ready. Your plan will help protect the health and safety of your community. Communication is an essential part of any successful public health response. Coordinate your planning activities with internal and external partners and stakeholders to help prepare your community for pandemic flu and achieve your emergency communication goals and objectives. Meet with your communication workgroup within 30 days after a flu pandemic ends. Debrief with workgroup members, partners, and stakeholders while they still remember events.

Readiness Resources

Pandemic Flu Planning Resources

CDC Pandemic Flu Planning Tools and Resources

■ Visit www.cdc.gov/npi for the latest information and resources about nonpharmaceutical interventions (NPIs)

■ Learn who may be at high risk for flu complications
http://www.cdc.gov/flu/about/disease/high_risk.htm

■ Community Mitigation Guidelines to Prevent Pandemic Influenza -